T0323467

MIRRORING BRAINS

GIACOMO RIZZOLATTI

and

CORRADO SINIGAGLIA

MIRRORING
BRAINS

how we understand others
from the inside

Translated by Frances Anderson

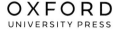

OXFORD
UNIVERSITY PRESS

OXFORD
UNIVERSITY PRESS

Great Clarendon Street, Oxford, OX2 6DP,
United Kingdom

Oxford University Press is a department of the University of Oxford.
It furthers the University's objective of excellence in research, scholarship,
and education by publishing worldwide. Oxford is a registered trade mark of
Oxford University Press in the UK and in certain other countries

The translation of this work has been funded by SEPS
Segretariato Europeo Per Le Pubblicazioni Scientifiche

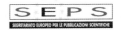

Via Val d'Aposa 7 - 40123 Bologna - Italy
seps@seps.it - www.seps.it

The moral rights of the authors have been asserted

First Edition published in 2023

Impression: 1

Published in the United States of America by Oxford University Press
198 Madison Avenue, New York, NY 10016, United States of America

British Library Cataloguing in Publication Data

Data available

Library of Congress Control Number: 2022946251

ISBN 978–0–19–887170–5

DOI: 10.1093/oso/9780198871705.001.0001

Printed in the UK by
Bell & Bain Ltd., Glasgow

PREFACE

At the end of the 1990s, Michael Arbib, mathematician and neuroscientist of the University of Southern California, dashed off a note to Giacomo Rizzolatti, 'We need to get a move on and write a book about the mirror neurons, because in a couple of years they'll be common knowledge and no one will be interested in them any more'. In the end, *we* wrote the book, although to be honest we took our time about it. *So quel che fai. Il cervello che agisce e i neuroni specchio* was published in Italian in 2006 with the English version following nine months later as *Mirrors in the Brain: How our minds share actions and emotions*. Contrary to Michael's prediction, however, mirror neurons did not lose their appeal and indeed still continue to be of interest to specialists and the general public alike, as is borne out by the success of that first book.

Over a decade has passed, and mirror neurons are still intriguing, even more so than before. Today we know that the mirror property—that property whereby a neuron responds both when we ourselves are engaged in a given behaviour and when we observe someone else engaged in it—is not an oddity of a handful of neurons in a very small portion of the premotor cortex, but characterizes a goodly part of our primate brain. A huge number of studies have contributed to substantially increasing our knowledge of how these neurons work and the role they might play, so our understanding of them is now much richer and multifaceted. These studies were not limited to the human brain; mirror neurons have also been identified in species very different from ours, such as marmosets, songbirds, rats, and bats. Given these developments, we decided to write another book together to present these new experimental findings and above all, explore their relative theoretical implications.

A main aim of *this book* is to show that the mirror property refers to a fundamental neuronal mechanism. Chapter 1 tackles this, describing the brain structures that currently are known to possess the mirror property and analysing the kind of mechanism they instantiate, so highlighting how mirror responses implicate a transformation of the sensory representations of the behaviour of others into the processes and representations that the observer would recruit if they were to behave in that self-same manner. As the anatomical and functional characteristics of the areas endowed with the mirror property can differ significantly from one brain structure to another, the incoming sensory representations as well as the outgoing processes and representations may vary. We will see that there are differences between the mirror responses recorded from the premotor and motor areas and, for example, those of the insula or the amygdala. In spite of these differences, however, all mirror responses embody a mechanism that transforms the processes and representations concerning a given behaviour we observe in other people into the processes and representations which are recruited when we produce that kind of behaviour ourselves. Given the nature and diffusion of the mirror responses, this mechanism appears to be a fundamental principle of the organization and functioning of the whole brain.

Chapter 2 focuses on *actions*, reviewing both the early and more recent studies. These suggest that mirror responses can involve a transformation of the sensory representations of the observed actions into the motor representations of their action goals similar to the representations that the observer would recruit if they were to plan and execute actions of that kind. We will show that this transformation is not connected to the merely visual aspects of the action being observed, nor to a specific sensory modality, but rather depends primarily on the capacity of the observer to *motorically* represent possible action goals. This is substantiated by the fact that the more this capacity is developed, the greater the possibility to *mirror* these goals when the actions are observed rather than executed.

One of the most fundamental discoveries in this field is that the mirror mechanism is not the prerogative of the cerebral areas concerned with the motor representation of action; it is also present in certain brain structures such as the insula, the amygdala and the cingulate gyrus that are known for being involved in producing motor and visceral responses characteristic of specific emotions such as, for instance, disgust and fear. Chapter 3 highlights that observing a grimace of disgust, a look of fear or a sonorous laugh triggers visceromotor representations similar to the representations that the observer would recruit if they were to experience the same kind of emotions themselves.

In Chapter 4 we argue that mirror responses may also concern what Daniel Stern defined as *vitality forms*. These forms characterize the dynamics of an action or an emotional reaction; for example, we speak about an *energetic* handshake, a *delicate* caress, a *violent* outburst of rage, a *hint* of a smile. Research in this field is still in the early stages, but there is enough data to suggest that there are indeed areas, such as the dorso-central portion of the insula, equipped with the mirror property for action-related vitality forms. Hence observing an action being executed gently or energetically prompts motor processes and representations that are similar to those the observer would recruit if they themselves were to execute that action with that particular vitality form.

Now that it has been ascertained that the mirror mechanism is present in various cerebral regions of different species and that, at least in the case of the primate brain, the transformations it entails can affect not only possible action goals but also emotional reactions and affective aspects, the question remains as to whether this mechanism has some form of cognitive function, and if so, what form this takes. Without a doubt, if not the most debated question of recent years, this is certainly one of the thorniest.

In the final two chapters, we develop and defend the theory that the mirror mechanism plays a distinctive role in understanding the actions, emotional reactions, and vitality forms we observe in others. In Chapter 5 we review the principal evidence that has emerged over the years in support of this theory, while in Chapter 6 we clarify the kind of understanding that mirror responses enable. In this regard, we have to distinguish between *basic* and *full-blown understanding*. While a *basic understanding* of an action can be reached by simply *identifying* its possible goal(s), a *full-blown understanding* requires a degree of *knowledge* of the states that motivated the execution of the action. The same holds true for emotions and vitality forms; it is one thing to *identify* the kind of emotion or the kind of vitality form displayed by an individual, it is quite another to *account* for why that individual, with their particular character, state of mind, sensitivity, and beliefs, experienced that kind of emotion or displayed that vitality form in that particular situation.

This allows us to take a first step towards clarifying in what sense the mirror mechanism plays a distinctive role in understanding other people's actions, emotions, and forms of vitality. In fact, we will argue and provide evidence that, all things being equal, mirror responses and their corresponding transformations are *sufficient* for a *basic understanding* of an action, emotional reaction, or a vitality form, while at the same time influencing the ability of the observer to *judge* them. This, of course, does not rule out the possibility that the actions, emotions, and vitality forms we observe in other people can be understood by processes and representations other than those evoked by mirror responses and their corresponding transformations. Indeed, drawing comparison with other forms of understanding will allow us to specify what kind of understanding of actions, emotions, and vitality forms we observe in other individuals can be attributed to mirror responses.

This leads us to introduce and discuss the notion of *understanding from the inside*, to which we have dedicated much thought in recent years and for which, in its initial form, we owe thanks to Marc Jeannerod. The phrase *from the inside* primarily refers to the fact the mirror mechanism would allow us to capture the 'intrinsic components' of an action we are observing, starting from its possible goals (Jeannerod, 2004). Mirror responses, in fact, would enable us to 'go inside' the observed action, by penetrating beyond the surface of its sensory aspects as we can capitalize on motor processes and representations similar to those we recruit when executing an action of that kind ourselves.

There is nothing strange or mysterious in all this. Anyone who is expert at activities involving particular motor skills, whether it be performing ballet, playing the piano, or playing basketball, is aware of having privileged access to the actions involved in these activities when they observe them being executed by others—and this even more so when the level of skills is similar to their own.

Not surprisingly, people who possess such skills understand the related actions more quickly and accurately than those who do not, as in understanding them, they deploy the same neuronal and representational resources they would use if they were actually executing the actions themselves. This is true to an even greater extent for emotions, as we will see when we discuss some emblematic cases of patients with lesions in brain structures with the mirror property.

The notion of *understanding from the inside* is susceptible to a second definition that in a certain sense integrates and expands the first. In fact, the understanding from the inside is not only characterized by the recruitment of representations usually involved in the carrying out of actions or emotional reactions, but also, and above all, by the fact that these representations can *shape* the experience of actions or emotions also when they are observed being performed or displayed by others. As we will see in Chapters 5 and 6, there is evidence to suggest that our experience of action or an emotion changes according to how it is represented motorically or viscerally. This applies not only to those actions and emotions we experience directly ourselves but also to those we observe in others. Assuming that this is indeed the case, understanding actions, emotions, and vitality forms of other people from the inside involves an experience of them, which, while undoubtedly differing from first-person action or emotion experience, will still share certain fundamental phenomenological aspects.

Apart from the obvious differences, executing an action or living an emotion and observing another person doing the same can be phenomenologically similar with respect to the kind of action or emotion in question. In some respects, what we experience when we observe others performing an action or living an emotion is what we experience when we perform that kind of action or live that kind of emotion ourselves. Mirroring the actions or emotions we observe in others enables us to share processes and representations but also, and most importantly, experiences; probably this is what makes it so special.

ACKNOWLEDGEMENTS

There are books that owe their existence to the efforts of more than one person; this is one such, and not just because it has two authors. Much of the data and many of the ideas presented in this volume are the result of years of research, with the significant contributions of many friends and colleagues. It would be impossible to mention them all, but we are grateful to each and every one of them. A particular vote of thanks is due to Michael Arbib, Luca Bonini, Stephen A. Butterfill, Luigi Cattaneo, Gergely Csibra, Luciano Fadiga, Pier Francesco Ferrari, Leonardo Fogassi, Vittorio Gallese, Alvin A. Goldman, Pierre Jacob, Christian Keysers, James Kilner, Roger Lemon, Guy A. Orban, Jean Michel Roy, Barry C. Smith, for having helped us to reflect on the mirror mechanism and its role in understanding the actions and emotions of others. A special mention is due to Daniel Stern, with whom a few years ago we started to explore the processes underlying the representation of our own vitality forms and those of others. We would also like to thank the team of the Claudio Munari Center for Epilepsy Surgery of Milan's Niguarda Hospital, in particular Ivana Maria Sartori and Giorgio Lo Russo, and Pietro Avanzini. A sincere thank you is due also to Fausto Caruana, especially for the section regarding disgust and laughter, and to Marzio Gerbella, who not only contributed a number of invaluable suggestions regarding the anatomical and functional characteristics of the various cerebral networks endowed with the mirror property, but also many of the illustrations contained in this volume.

Finally, our heartfelt gratitude goes to the late Giulio Giorello for his constant and unwavering support and to Raffaello Cortina who particularly desired us to write this book; to Mariella Agostinelli for the grace and competence with which she monitored our progress, and Giorgio Catalano and Martina Scarpa for their invaluable editorial assistance and attention to detail.

CONTENTS

ABBREVIATIONS

ACC	Anterior cingulate cortex
AI	Anterior insula
AIP	Anterior Intraparietal area
aMCC	Anterior middle cingulate cortex
cTBS	Continuous thetaburst stimulation
DCI	Dorso-central insula
EBA	Extrastriate body area
EEG	Electroencephalogram
ERP	Event related potentials
FEF	Frontal eye field
fMRI	Functional magnetic resonance imaging
IPL	Inferior parietal lobe
LIP	Lateral intraparietal area
MI/F$_1$	Primary motor cortex
MCC	Middle cingulate cortex
MEG	Magnetoencephalography
MEP	Motor evoked potential
MT	Medial temporal cortex
pACC	Pregenual anterior cingulate cortex
PAG	Periaqueductal gray
PCC	Posterior cingulate cortex
PET	Positron emission tomography
pMCC	Posterior middle cingulate cortex
PMd/F$_2$	Dorsal premotor cortex

PMv	Ventral premotor cortex
Pre-SMA/F6	Pre-supplementary motor area
pSTS	Posterior superior temporal sulcus
RSC	Retrosplenial cingulate cortex
rTMS	Repetitive transcranial magnetic stimulation
SII	Secondary somatosensory cortex
sACC	Subgenual anterior cingulate cortex
SMA/MII/F3	Supplementary motor area
STS	Superior temporal sulcus
TMS	Transcranial magnetic stimulation
TPJ	Temporo-parietal junction
VIP	Ventral intraparietal area
vPCC	Ventral posterior cingulate cortex

CHAPTER 1

A MIRRORING BRAIN

Over the years, several cerebral areas have been found to possess the mirror property. In this chapter we will map those areas and will show that far from characterizing a single brain network, this property can be considered a fundamental principle of the functioning of the entire nervous system. A neuron is said to be a *mirror neuron* if it fires both when an individual displays a kind of behaviour and also when they observe the same kind of behaviour being displayed by others. In the following pages, we will begin with the first studies carried out in the 1990s by a group of researchers at the University of Parma that led to the discovery of mirror neurons in the premotor cortex of the macaque. We will then focus on the subsequent research that revealed the presence of mirror neurons in other areas of the frontal, parietal, and prefrontal lobes. We will also review, albeit briefly, the vast literature that contributed to individuating human brain areas endowed with the mirror property not only in the frontal and the parietal lobes, but also in brain structures such as the insula, the amygdala, and the cingulate gyrus. Lastly, we will look at research done on other species such as marmosets, birds, rats, and bats, so as to offer an initial characterization of the mechanism underlying what can justifiably be called a *mirroring brain*.

Mirroring Brains. Giacomo Rizzolatti and Corrado Sinigaglia, Oxford University Press. © Oxford University Press 2023. DOI: 10.1093/oso/9780198871705.003.0001

Mirror Neurons in the Macaque

Early data

For a long time it was thought that the *agranular* frontal cortex in the macaque brain, corresponding to Brodmann areas 4 and 6 and classically considered as the motor cortex, was composed of two functionally distinct areas: the primary motor cortex, characterized by a complete and fine-grained representation of movements, and the supplementary motor cortex in which the representation of movement is less defined.[1]

Today, mainly due to the work of Massimo Matelli and colleagues at the University of Parma, we know that the agranular frontal cortex is composed of seven *anatomically* separate areas, identified by the letter F (standing for Frontal) followed by an Arabic numeral from 1 to 7 (Matelli et al., 1985; Matelli et al., 1991; Belmalih et al., 2007). F1 refers to the primary motor cortex (sometimes indicated as MI) and corresponds roughly to Brodmann area 4. Brodmann area 6, on the other hand, is divided into three main regions (mesial, dorsal, and ventral), which in turn are divided into the rostral (anterior) and caudal (posterior) parts. The mesial region is composed of areas F3 (SMA) and F6 (pre-SMA), while the dorsal region (the premotor dorsal cortex, PMd) includes areas F2

---

[1] Whoever is familiar with neurophysiological handbooks will certainly remember Clinton Woolsey's famous *simiunculus* and Wilder Penfield's equally well-known *homunculus,* mapped in the mid-1900s in monkeys and humans, respectively, by electrically stimulating the motor cortex with macroelectrodes positioned on the surface. Both identified two motor areas: the primary (MI/F1) and supplementary (SMA, sometimes also indicated as MII/F3) motor areas, with a complete representation of movement, in greater detail in MI and more roughly in SMA. For further reading on this subject, see Rizzolatti and Sinigaglia (2008).

(whose proper denomination is PMd) and F7 (pre-PMd) and lastly, the ventral region (ventral premotor cortex, PMv), which consists of areas F4 and F5 (Fig. 1.1).

Since the mid-1980s, Giacomo Rizzolatti, Maurizio Gentilucci, and colleagues at the University of Parma have been systematically studying the *functional* properties of the motor areas, particularly area F5, registering the action potentials of single neurons (Gentilucci et al., 1988; Rizzolatti et al., 1988). The neuronal activity was recorded while the macaques were freely executing various actions, all present in their own motor repertoire, such as picking

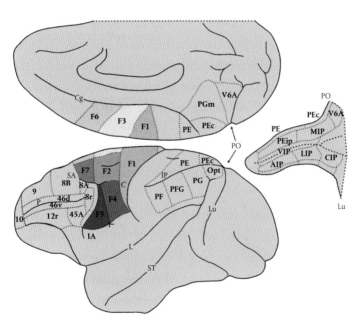

Fig. 1.1 Mesial and lateral views of the macaque brain showing the anatomical and functional parcellation of the agranular frontal cortex.

Abbreviations: IA = inferior arcuate sulcus, C = central sulcus, Cg = cingulate sulcus, IP = intraparietal sulcus, L = lateral fissure or fissure of Silvius, Lu = lunate sulcus, P = principal sulcus, PO = parieto-occipital sulcus, SA = superior arcuate sulcus ST = superior temporal sulcus.

up a piece of food, holding it in their hand, lifting it to their mouth but also cracking a nut or swatting an object away. Sometimes the experimenters would lay out a variety of visual stimuli, pieces of food or objects of different shape, size, and orientation, placing them close to or far from the animal. They would also execute actions in front of the animal that were very similar to those the animal itself was accustomed to performing.

This approach turned out to be particularly successful, facilitating an ethological study of area F5 (but not only!) neuron responses, and the discovery of properties that would probably never have emerged if the neuronal activity had been recorded exclusively while the animal was executing predetermined and highly stereotypical movements. The first to be identified was a functional property that characterizes most F5 neurons: in many cases, their firing during the execution of a given action represents the *goal* of said action, and not simply this or that single movement somehow involved in the achievement of that goal (Rizzolatti et al., 1988). As we will see in Chapter 2 (pp. 40–48), this property is particularly important in the definition of the role and functions of motor processes and representations as we understand them today.

A second discovery was that a number of F5 neurons that fired while the macaque was executing an action such as grasping a small object, a sunflower seed for example, between the index finger and the thumb, also fired when the animal was presented with a piece of food or any other object that could be picked up with that kind of grip. This occurred regardless of whether the object was actually grasped or not (Rizzolatti et al., 1988; Murata et al., 1997). These neurons, characterized by congruent motor and visual responses, are known as *canonical neurons*.

The third and most important discovery was made by a group of researchers led by Giacomo Rizzolatti, including Luciano Fadiga, Leonardo Fogassi, Vittorio Gallese and, in the early days, Giuseppe di Pellegrino: a number of F5 neurons that fired while the macaque was executing a specific action also fired when it saw the researcher executing the same kind of action, whereas the mere presentation of visual stimuli showing food or various objects failed to evoke a response (di Pellegrino et al., 1992; Gallese et al., 1996; Rizzolatti, Fadiga, Gallese et al., 1996). These neurons were given the name *mirror neurons*. Fig. 1.2 shows the activity of one such neuron: the lower panel (B) shows the discharges of the neuron while the macaque is grasping the food, whereas the upper panel (A) shows the discharges of the same neuron while the macaque observes the

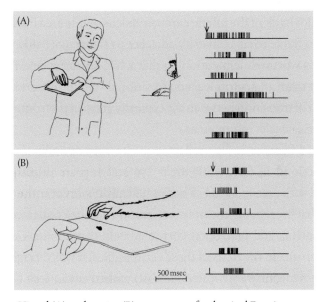

Fig. 1.2 Visual (A) and motor (B) responses of a classical F5 mirror neuron (di Pellegrino et al., 1992).

researcher executing the same kind of action. The congruence of the neuronal discharge profiles in the two conditions, respectively of executing the action and of observing it, is of particular importance.

Mirror neurons in the frontal lobe

Area F5 is located in the anterior portion of the premotor ventral cortex (PMv). Giuseppe Luppino and colleagues have shown that this area is not anatomically homogeneous, consisting as it does of three subareas that are cytoarchitectonically distinct, differing from each other in the organization and layout of the various types of cells: convexity F5 (F5c), posterior F5 (F5p), and anterior F5 (F5a) (Belmalih et al., 2009). Areas F5p and F5a are located on the posterior bank of the inferior arcuate sulcus, while area F5c is situated on the cortical convexity adjacent to the arcuate sulcus (Fig. 1.3). It is worthwhile mentioning that while areas F5p and F5c are similar from an anatomical and functional standpoint, area F5a is an area of transition between the typically *granular* prefrontal areas and the *agranular* motor areas.

This difference is also reflected in the correspondent cortical connections: in fact, while areas F5c and F5p are directly connected with area F1, area F5a has practically no direct connections with that area, being the only subarea of F5 to be connected with the ventrolateral prefrontal cortex (Matelli et al., 1986; Gerbella et al., 2011). On the basis of these early studies, it was thought that mirror neurons were located (almost) exclusively in area F5c and canonical neurons in area F5p. However, a later study (Bonini et al., 2014) showed that mirror and canonical neurons are to be found

6

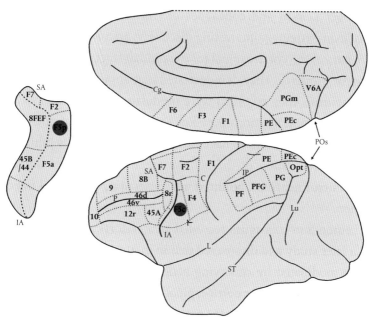

Fig. 1.3 Lateral and mesial views of the macaque brain. The hidden areas of the arcuate sulcus are shown on the left. The two sub-areas of F5, that according to currently available data have the mirror property, are highlighted in red.

Abbreviations: IA = inferior arcuate sulcus, C = central sulcus, Cg = cingulate sulcus, IP = intraparietal sulcus, L = lateral fissure or fissure of Silvius, Lu = lunate sulcus, P = principal sulcus, POs = parieto-occipital sulcus, SA = superior arcuate sulcus, ST = superior temporal sulcus.

in both areas, with a slight predominance of mirror neurons in area F5c and canonical neurons in area F5p (Fig. 1.3). Interestingly, this study also described a set of neurons with both canonical and mirror properties. Indeed, these neurons (known as *canonical-mirror neurons*) discharge while a given action is being executed on a target object with a specific shape and size, when someone is observed executing the action (mirror property) or again at the sight of a target object, with that specific shape and size (canonical property).

Roger Lemon and colleagues of University College London made an extremely interesting discovery: area F5p neurons that are part of the corticospinal (or pyramidal) tract may exhibit the mirror property. They demonstrated that approximately 50% of the neurons they recorded were modulated by the observation of other people's actions (Kraskov et al., 2009). About one-third of the neurons found to have the mirror property was inhibited during observation of the actions executed by others (inhibitory mirror neurons), but fired while executing the same kind of action.

Lemon and colleagues recorded area F1 corticospinal neurons in a later study and discovered that in many cases their activities were modulated by observing actions executed by others (Fig. 1.4). As happens in the corticospinal tract that starts in area F5, in one part of these neurons the response increased when observing actions performed by others, but was inhibited in another part (Vigneswaran et al., 2013). Nevertheless, the mirror responses of the area F1 corticospinal neurons were much weaker than the homologous F5 neurons, which would explain why no significant mirror activity was found in area F1 in the initial recordings (Gallese et al., 1996; Fogassi et al., 2001).

Mirror neurons have also been described in the dorsal premotor cortex (PMd), in area F2 (Fig. 1.4). Paul Cisek and John Kalaska at the University of Montreal did in fact find F2 neurons that fired both when their macaques correctly guided a cursor to point to a target previously indicated between two possible options and when the animals observed the experimenter moving the cursor to the correct target. When the experimenter moved the cursor to the correct target, the macaques received some juice as a reward.

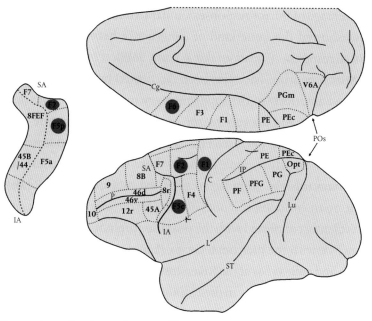

Fig. 1.4 Lateral and mesial views of the macaque brain. The frontal areas that have mirror properties (according to currently available data) are highlighted in red.

Abbreviations: IA = inferior arcuate sulcus, C = central sulcus, Cg = cingulate sulcus, IP = intraparietal sulcus, L = lateral fissure or fissure of Silvius, Lu = lunate sulcus, P = principal sulcus, POs = parieto-occipital sulcus, SA = superior arcuate sulcus, ST = superior temporal sulcus.

It was interesting to see that the neuronal activity was practically identical at both the individual and population levels in both conditions (Cisek & Kalaska, 2004). Later experiments using similar tasks identified mirror responses in area F2 as well as in area F1 (Tkach et al., 2007; Dushanova & Donoghue, 2010). Lastly, a recent study examined the activity of F2 neurons during the execution and observation of grasping actions similar to those typically used to investigate F5 mirror neurons. Not only did F2 neurons show a percentage of mirror responses similar to that of F5 neurons, they also showed the same kind of congruence between motor and visual responses (Papadourakis & Raos, 2018).

Mirror neurons have also been discovered in area F6, which is located anteriorly to the supplementary motor area proper (area F3 or SMA) and for this reason is often indicated as pre-SMA (Matsuzaka et al., 1992; see Fig. 1.4). In spite of its fundamentally agranular structure, area F6 does show transitional character-istics towards the granular areas of the prefrontal lobe (Matelli et al., 1991). In addition, it does not project directly to area F1 as it is prevalently connected with the posterior premotor areas, and like area F5a, with the prefrontal cortex (Luppino et al., 1993). Masaki Isoda and colleagues at the Riken Institute recorded F6 neuron ac-tivity in two macaques; in their study, the two monkeys each had a button they had to push in turn, depending on the choice made by the other (Yoshida et al., 2011). In this study the authors identified three kinds of neurons: the so-called *self*-neurons that fired only while the action was being executed; the *other*-neurons that fired only when observing the other macaque executing the action; and, finally, the neurons that fired in both conditions, thus exhib-iting the property that characterizes mirror neurons. Luca Bonini and colleagues at the University of Parma obtained similar results from a classic Go/NoGo experiment with macaques, consisting in reaching for and grasping different-sized objects or watching the hand of an experimenter, seated behind the animal, performing the same task (Livi et al., 2019). In this study too, the authors found neurons that fired only when the macaques themselves executed the action of reaching and grasping, others that fired only when they watched the experimenter doing the reaching and grasping, and those which fired in both conditions (mirror neurons).

Mirror neurons in the parietal lobe

A number of other single cell recordings have demonstrated that mirror neurons are also present in the inferior parietal lobe (IPL). The first studies recorded mirror neurons from the IPL convexity, in particular from the PF and PFG areas (Gallese et al., 2002; Fogassi et al., 2005; Rozzi et al., 2008), while subsequent studies found them in the anterior intraparietal area (AIP) (Pani et al., 2014; Maeda et al., 2015), where the presence of visuomotor neurons with functional characteristics not unlike the F5 canonical neurons had been previously reported (Murata et al., 2000; see Fig. 1.5).

For many years it was thought that the function of the posterior parietal lobe was mainly, if not exclusively, to associate and integrate sensory information into 'percepts' that could then be used when exploring the surrounding world, both as a guide to action and as a basis for categorization. This changed however when it was discovered that a significant portion of the posterior parietal areas is not only somatotopically organized, but also contains neurons with undeniably motor properties (Hyvärinen, 1981; Andersen, 1987; Mountcastle, 1995; Sakata et al., 1995). Today we know that the posterior parietal lobe is composed of a plurality of nodes connected to various centres, each with specific functional characteristics. For the purposes of this book, it is useful to remember that the area denominated as PFG has strong connections with the neighbouring areas of the inferior parietal lobule (PF, PG, AIP, and VIP), the adjacent parietal operculum, the insula, the premotor ventral areas (particularly area F5) and the prefrontal lobe, notably area 46. The AIP area is densely connected with the adjacent parietal areas (PF, PFG, PG, LIP, and VIP), vast sectors of the inferior temporal cortex, the insula, area F5, and the prefrontal

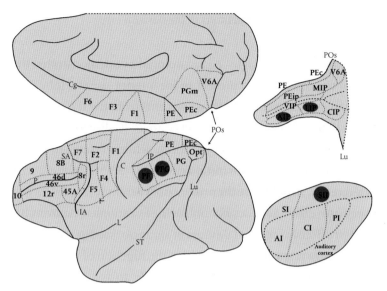

Fig. 1.5 Lateral and mesial views of the macaque brain. The parietal areas that have mirror properties (according to currently available data) are highlighted in red. The hidden areas of the intraparietal sulcus (top) and lateral sulcus (bottom) are shown on the right.

Abbreviations: IA = inferior arcuate sulcus, C = central sulcus, Cg = cingulate sulcus, IP = intraparietal sulcus, L = lateral fissure or fissure of Silvius, Lu = lunate sulcus, P = principal sulcus, POs = parieto-occipital sulcus, SA = superior arcuate sulcus, ST = superior temporal sulcus.

ventrolateral cortex, in particular areas 12r and 46v (Luppino et al., 1999; Borra et al., 2008; Borra et al., 2011; Gerbella et al., 2013; Lanzilotto et al., 2019).

Mirror neurons have also been found in other two parietal areas: the ventral intraparietal (VIP) and the lateral intraparietal (LIP) areas (see Fig. 1.5). In addition to its visual neurons, the VIP area contains bimodal neurons that are activated not only by somatosensory stimuli, but also by visual stimuli, provided that these are close to the skin and the tactile receptive field (Colby et al., 1993; Duhamel et al., 1998). Akira Murata and his collaborators at the Kinki University of Osaka ran an interesting experiment on macaques, during which they discovered that not only did some VIP bimodal neurons fire when a visual stimulus was brought into the animal's proximity, but also when it was brought close to the experimenter, even if the latter was at a fair distance from the monkey (Ishida et al., 2010). It is important to note that if the experimenter was not physically present, these VIP neurons did not react to visual stimuli shown at that same distance. In addition, the VIP neuron visual responses were congruent, i.e. if the visual receptive field of the VIP neuron was close to the macaque's nose, the neuron also fired when the visual stimulus was shown close to the experimenter's nose.

The LIP area is situated in the posterior part of the IPL lateral bank (see Fig. 1.5); it receives significant input from the visual areas and is connected to the frontal eye fields (FEF), which explains why many LIP neurons fire during saccadic eye movements as well as in the presence of visual stimuli (Andersen et al., 1997; Colby & Goldberg, 1999). Michael Platt and colleagues at Duke University, working with macaques, took recordings from the LIP area during tasks that included executing a rapid saccadic movement in a given direction and observing a static image of another macaque looking either in the same or in the opposite direction (Shepherd et al., 2009). They found that a number of LIP neurons fired both when the macaque looked in a given direction and when it observed the static image of the macaque looking in the same direction.

Lastly, mirror neurons were individuated in the secondary somatosensory cortex (SII) (see Fig. 1.5). Sayaka Hihara and colleagues at the Riken Institute recorded the activity of single neurons from the SII and neighbouring areas while visual stimuli representing objects, hand movements, and grasping actions were being presented (Hihara et al., 2015). Their results showed that there were neurons in this area that responded selectively both to objects within hand's reach and to the observation of movements without a specific goal, but what was even more interesting, they responded to actual grasping actions.

Mirror neurons in the prefrontal lobe

Mirror neurons have very recently been found in the prefrontal lobe. Stefano Rozzi and colleagues at the University of Parma have recorded the activity of single neurons in the frontal ventrolateral cortex, notably in the rostral portion of area 12 (12r), the ventral portion of area 46 (46v) and area 45A (see Fig. 1.6), of macaques watching a video of arm and hand movements, some of which had the goal of grasping food or some other item, others simply of moving objects (Simone et al., 2017). Their results show that in a good percentage of the recorded neurons the responses were selective for the observation of reaching and grasping actions executed by another macaque or by an experimenter. These results are in line with the findings from an earlier fMRI study conducted by Guy Orban and colleagues at the University of Leuven; these authors reported activation of areas 45A and 46 when the macaque was shown grasping actions (Nelissen et al., 2005). Of particular interest is the fact that a number of the recorded neurons responded also when reaching and grasping actions were being executed, proof that they too have the mirror property (Simone et al., 2015).

Finally, mirror neurons have also been found in area 9 (Fig. 1.6), where they have been recorded responding to a head-rotation

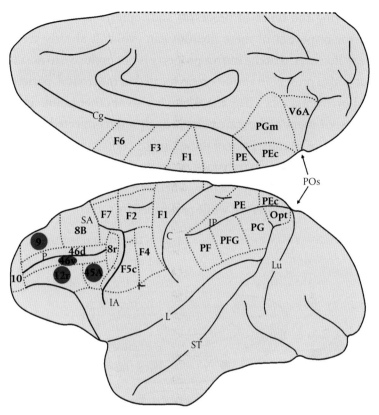

Fig. 1.6 Lateral and mesial views of the macaque brain. The prefrontal areas that have mirror properties (according to currently available data) are highlighted in red.

Abbreviations: IA = inferior arcuate sulcus, C = central sulcus, Cg = cingulate sulcus, IP = intraparietal sulcus, L = lateral fissure or fissure of Silvius, Lu = lunate sulcus, P = principal sulcus, POs = parieto-occipital sulcus, SA = superior arcuate sulcus, ST = superior temporal sulcus.

movement, both when this was executed by the macaque and when the animal was observing the movement being executed by an experimenter (Lanzilotto et al., 2017).

In the next chapter we will have the opportunity of analysing the functional properties of the mirror neurons in detail and specifying the types of processes and representations that the mirror responses of these neurons can evoke. It already seems clear, however, that the mirror property is not exclusive to area F5 but is also present in various areas located in the frontal, parietal, and prefrontal lobes (Fig. 1.7). There is also another point: as we have seen, many of these areas are strongly interconnected, producing a set of circuits. Each of these circuits contributes, according to its specific functional characteristics, to the processing of information regarding a given action, whether it is being performed in person or being observed while performed by someone else.

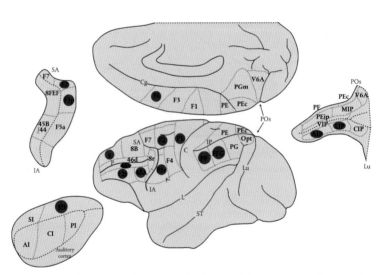

Fig. 1.7 Lateral and mesial views of the brain of the macaque; all areas that have mirror properties (according to currently available data) are highlighted in red.

Abbreviations: IA = inferior arcuate sulcus, C = central sulcus, Cg = cingulate sulcus, IP = intraparietal sulcus, L = lateral fissure or fissure of Silvius, Lu = lunate sulcus, P = principal sulcus, POs = parieto-occipital sulcus, SA = superior arcuate sulcus, ST = superior temporal sulcus.

Mirror Neurons in Humans

Early data

Immediately after the discovery of mirror neurons in area F5 of the macaque, studies were conducted to explore the possibility that these neurons could also be present in humans. A number of techniques were used in these studies, ranging from Positron Emission Tomography (PET) and functional Magnetic Resonance Imaging (fMRI) to Electroencephalography (EEG), Magnetoencephalography (MEG), and Transcranial Magnetic Stimulation (TMS).

The first of these studies dates back to the mid-1990s. It was conducted by Giacomo Rizzolatti with the collaboration of Ferruccio Fazio, Daniela Perani, and colleagues of Milan's San Raffaele Hospital, which at that time was one of the few places in Italy to possess PET technology. Using this technology, they investigated whether observing another person executing an action would activate the observer's own motor areas. The most important finding was that when a person lying in the scanner watched an experimenter executing grasping actions, the caudal portion of their inferior frontal gyrus became active (Rizzolatti, Fadiga, Matelli et al., 1996). Giacomo Rizzolatti and colleagues obtained analogous results in a study carried out with Scott Grafton's group at the University of Southern California, Santa Barbara (Grafton et al., 1996).

An fMRI study conducted by Giacomo Rizzolatti with the collaboration of Hans Freud and colleagues at the University of Düsseldorf at the Jülich Research Center, directed at the time by Karl Zilles, contributed to obtaining a more complete picture of the premotor areas that are involved in observing action (Buccino et al., 2001). The comparison between the observation of actions executed with various effectors (hand, mouth, and foot) revealed the existence of a somatotopy in the premotor area and the inferior parietal lobule, corresponding to the somatotopical organization described in clinical neurology.

EEG and MEG studies have also provided evidence supporting the presence of mirror neurons in humans. EEG studies record spontaneous electrical activity in the brain and classify the various rhythms according to the wave frequencies. At rest, the alpha (α) rhythm (8–12 Hz) prevails in the posterior regions of the cerebral cortex, while the so-called desynchronized rhythms, i.e. those with high frequency and low voltage, are dominant in the frontal lobe. There is also another rhythm known as mu (μ), similar to the α rhythm, which is frequently observed in the central regions of the cerebral cortex, corresponding to the motor areas. The μ rhythm is present as long as the motor system is at rest: an active movement desynchronizes it. Vilayanur Ramachandran and colleagues at the University of California of San Diego were the first to demonstrate the desynchronization of the μ rhythm while their participants were observing the actions of others (Altschuler et al., 1997, 2000). Catherine Barthélémy and colleagues at the University of Tours carried out a similar study, demonstrating that the observation of leg or finger movements was accompanied by the desynchronization of the μ rhythm, which did not occur when their participants were shown a visual stimulus depicting a moving object (Cochin et al., 1999).

Analogous results were obtained from a series of research studies using MEG, a technique that analyses the electrical activity of the brain from recordings of the magnetic fields it generates. Like EEG, this technique measures the temporal dynamics of the activation of the various cortical areas involved in a given task. Using MEG, Riita Hari and colleagues at the University of Helsinki brought to light a desynchronization of the μ rhythm in the precentral cortex both when their participants were handling an object themselves and when they watched another person handling it. They did not find this desynchronization when the participants were observing moving objects (Hari et al., 1998). At a later date, Hari's team demonstrated how observing grasping actions activates not only the visual areas but also the caudal portion of the left inferior frontal gyrus, the left primary motor area, and finally the primary contralateral motor area. This pattern was identical to that observed when the same kind of actions were being executed, excluding the visual areas of course (Nishitani & Hari, 2000).

A number of TMS studies provided further convincing evidence that the human motor system is endowed with the mirror property. TMS is a non-invasive technique that stimulates the nervous system; by applying a magnetic stimulus to the primary motor cortex with the appropriate intensity, motor evoked potentials (referred to as MEP) can be recorded in the muscles of effectors such as hands and feet. Luciano Fadiga and colleagues at the University of Parma recorded MEPs induced by the stimulation of the left primary motor cortex in muscles of the right hands and arms of their participants, who were asked to watch an experimenter grasping objects with her hand (Fadiga et al., 1995). As a control condition, the participants were asked to look at a pinpoint of light and report if they had noticed it dimming in intensity. While they were watching the experimenter grasping, their MEPs increased in the muscles they would have used had they been doing the grasping themselves; there was no comparable effect in the control condition. Interestingly, by using the 'double-pulse' TMS technique, Antonio Strafella and Tomàš Paus demonstrated that the increase in MEPs while observing an action is the result of a cortico-cortical activation with the primary motor cortex being triggered by the premotor cortex (Strafella & Paus, 2000).

The parieto-frontal network

The numerous brain-imaging studies carried out in the following years made it possible to draw up a detailed description of a network of parietal and frontal areas that have the mirror property. A number of meta-analyses combining data from several hundreds of studies (Caspers et al., 2010; Grosbras et al., 2012; Molenberghs et al., 2012), show that the inferior parietal lobule (IPL), the ventral premotor cortex (PMv), and the caudal sector of the inferior frontal gyrus are the principal nodes of the parieto-frontal network involved in grasping actions (Fig. 1.8).

It is important to keep in mind that the great majority of the studies involved in the meta-analyses only took the activation of the areas mentioned above into consideration while actions were being observed. This is understandable because it is difficult to study movements in a scanner without producing artefacts due to modifications of the magnetic field. A few studies, however, were able to overcome this difficulty and to explore the activation of the parieto-frontal motor areas both when the participants were executing certain actions themselves and when they were observing actions being executed. One example is the study run by Valeria Gazzola and Christian Keysers at the University of Groningen, who asked their participants to observe actions being executed,

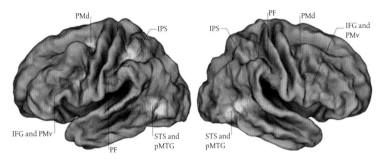

Fig. 1.8 Parietal and frontal areas endowed with the mirror property revealed by a meta-analysis of studies on observation of grasping actions, including the activations linked to both the hand and the mouth.

Abbreviations: IFG = inferior frontal gyrus, PMd = dorsal premotor cortex, pMTG = posterior portion of the medial temporal gyrus, PMv = ventral premotor cortex, STS = superior temporal sulcus (adapted from Caspers et al., 2010).

mainly manually, and then execute the actions themselves. After analysing each individual participant's unsmoothed data, they found that there were some voxels in the nodes of the parieto-frontal network that were common to the actions observed and to those executed (Gazzola & Keysers, 2009).

In a later study, Keysers and colleagues recorded the EEG and BOLD signals simultaneously during the execution and observation of manual actions (Arnstein et al., 2011). The purpose of the study was twofold: on the one hand, to demonstrate that the suppression of the μ rhythm correlates with the BOLD signal, so as to be able to consider both the markers equivalent in terms of their functional significance; on the other, to improve the previous analysis, so as to precisely identify the regions that are activated both when actions are executed and their execution is being observed. The results showed that the μ rhythm covaried with the intensity of the BOLD signal in those regions that typically have the mirror property.

The studies that have been mentioned here were mainly conducted on grasping acts, mostly involving the distal limbs. However, there were others that explored the existence of motor areas, endowed with the mirror property, encoding proximal movements of the upper limbs. Flavia Filimon and colleagues at the University of California of San Diego studied reaching movements in three conditions: execution, observation, and imagination. They found that activations overlapped in the parietal lobule and the dorsal premotor cortex in all three conditions (Filimon et al., 2007; see Fig. 1.9).

There are two points here that are worthy of mention: first, mirror responses to reaching actions are located more dorsally with respect to mirror responses to manipulative actions; second, the strong similarity of these data to the findings in the literature regarding the anatomical and functional characteristics of the

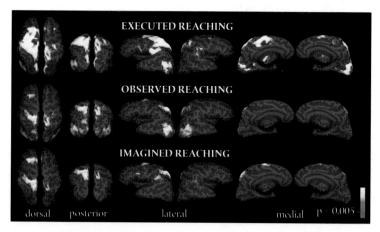

Fig. 1.9 Cortical activations during the execution, observation, and imagination of reaching actions. Note the overlapping of the activations in the dorsal premotor cortex and the superior parietal lobule in the three conditions (adapted from Filimon et al., 2007).

22

parietal and dorsal premotor cortices that are considered to play a key role in controlling proximal movements in non-human primates. In a more recent study, Cinzia di Dio and colleagues showed that the superior parietal lobule and the dorsal premotor cortex became active while observing biological motion being carried out by a biological effector (an arm) or a non-biological object (an arrow). However, there was no activation in the superior parietal and dorsal premotor areas while the subjects were observing objects moving towards a given position in space, following the same trajectory but with non-biological movement (Di Dio et al., 2013). Guy Orban and colleagues at the University of Leuven compared observations of two different kinds of action: manipulation and climbing. Their results confirmed the inferior parietal/ventral premotor activation while observing manipulative actions, while to the contrary, when their participants were observing someone climbing, the activation was more dorsal, thus extending to the superior parietal and the dorsal premotor cortices (Abdollahi et al., 2013).

When we observe actions being executed by other humans, our medial frontal areas activate just as those of macaques do. Roy Mukamel and colleagues at the University of California of Los Angeles conducted one of the rare studies in which human neurons have been recorded, examining the responses of the Supplementary Motor Area (SMA) and pre-SMA during execution and observation of grasping actions (Mukamel et al., 2010). Their results showed that, while a significant proportion of neurons fired exclusively during the execution or observation of a given grasping action, a number fired in both conditions. What is particularly interesting is that a subset of these neurons showed excitation during the execution of an action and inhibition while it was being observed.

Lastly, just as in the macaque, mirror responses have been found in the human secondary somatosensory cortex (SII). For example, Christian Keysers and colleagues (2004) demonstrated that the activation of the SII, which was stimulated by getting their participants to observe a person being touched, overlapped, at least partially, with the activation recorded when they were touched themselves. Very similar results were obtained by Susan Blakemore and colleagues of University College London, who found not only that the SII was activated while observing a person being touched, but that the activation was much more pronounced in sufferers of visual tactile synaesthesia (Blakemore et al., 2005). Finally, in an FMRI study conducted a few years later, Zarinah Agnew and Richard Wise showed that the SII responded also when observing actions being executed by others (Agnew & Wise, 2008). Comparing the activations of the parietal operculum while performing and observing finger movements, these authors discovered a clear overlapping in the lateral portion of the SII, demonstrating that is endowed with the mirror property.

The insula

From the very early years of this century, studies using brain imaging, electrostimulation, and intracortical recording have shown that the mirror property is not limited to the parietal and frontal areas involved in representing action, but is also present in cortical areas and centres underlying various emotional or affective behaviours. One of these centres is the insula.

The insula, triangular in shape and divided into anterior and posterior sections by a central sulcus, is connected to various other cortical areas and sends descending connections to structures that are fundamental for displaying emotional reactions, such as the hypothalamus, the periaqueductal gray (PAG) and the centromedial nuclei of the amygdala (Gothard & Hoffman, 2010). Three main regions, anterior, dorso-central (with a caudal extension) and ventral, have been functionally individuated by applying cortical microstimulation to awake non-human primates. The anterior insula contains a mosaic of bucco-facial behaviours, shifting gradually from ingestive actions, which are more dorsal, to emotional reactions (e.g. disgust), that are more ventral. The dorso-central insula contains a sensorimotor field that shows functional similarities with the contiguous portion of the parietal lobe Finally, stimulation of the ventral insula evokes affiliative gestures (Caruana et al., 2011; Jezzini et al., 2012).

Although the human insula is much larger than that of the macaque, its anatomical and functional organization appears to be similar (Kurth et al., 2010). It is composed of four main and distinct functional fields: sensorimotor, gustatory-olfactory, social-emotional, and cognitive. The sensorimotor field is situated in the dorso-central insula; there is a similar field in the macaque. The gustatory-olfactory field corresponds to the positive and negative ingestive sectors of the macaque's brain, while the social-emotional field is located in the ventral portion of the insula. Finally, the cognitive field is extremely heterogeneous and is involved in attentional and working memory processes (Mayer et al., 2007; Sörös et al., 2007; Corbetta et al., 2008). It has been hypothesized that this field is linked to internal language (Vignolo et al., 1986), which might explain why the functions that have been attributed to it are so diverse. No such field has been identified in the macaque.

fMRI studies have shown that the anterior insula (AI), or at least a part of it, is characterized by the mirror property. In particular, they have shown that when we see someone grimacing in disgust, this activates an area of AI very similar to that which is activated when we experience repulsive tastes or odours ourselves (Wicker et al., 2003; Jabbi et al., 2007; see also Gallese et al., 2004). Pierre Krolak-Salmon and colleagues (2003) obtained analogous results when recording event-related potentials (ERP) from the AI of patients with drug-refractory temporal lobe epilepsy while they were observing expressions of disgust on other people's faces.

A series of recent fMRI studies has individuated mirror responses in the dorso-central section of the insula (DCI) (Fig. 1.10). Observing actions imbued with a specific affective significance—or, more precisely, a specific *vitality form*—*provoked* activation of the

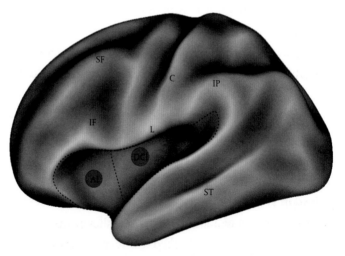

Fig. 1.10 Portions of the insula that currently appear to have the mirror property, illustrated on a standard brain generated by Caret software.

Abbreviations: SF = superior frontal sulcus, IF = inferior frontal sulcus, C = central sulcus, IP = intraparietal sulcus, L = lateral fissure, ST = superior temporal sulcus.

DCI in the observer's brain similar to that which occurred when an action with that same vitality form was being executed as opposed to being observed (Di Cesare et al., 2014; Di Cesare et al., 2015).

The amygdala

The mirror property has also been found in the amygdala, a complex telencephalic, almond-shaped structure composed of thirteen nuclei situated in the anterior portion of the medial temporal lobe. As well as being connected to the temporal and prefrontal regions (Amaral & Price, 1984; Gerbella et al., 2014), the amygdala projects to subcortical areas such as the medial hypothalamus, the lateral region of the PAG, the locus coeruleus, and parabrachial nuclei that control the responses of the nervous system linked to defensive fight-or-flight behaviour (Moga & Gray, 1985; Price et al., 1987; An et al., 1998; Motta et al., 2009).

Several brain-imaging studies have shown that the amygdala activates when people see faces expressing fear (Morris et al., 1996; Phillips et al., 1997, 1998). Similar data were also obtained from a series of intracranial ERP recordings obtained from patients with drug-refractory temporal lobe epilepsy while looking at pictures of faces with expressions of fear (Krolak-Salmon et al., 2004; Sato et al., 2011; Méndez-Bértolo et al., 2016) (Fig. 1.11).

Although these studies focused exclusively on what happens while observing fearful expressions on other people's faces, the stimulation of the amygdala in patients provokes physiological and motor reactions typically associated with the experience of fear (Meletti et al., 2006; Inman et al., 2018). This indicates that the amygdala (or some of its nuclei) has the mirror property, as it is

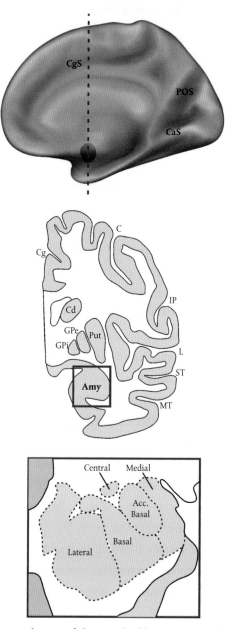

Fig. 1.11 Left: a mesial view of the standard brain generated by Caret software, showing the position of the amygdala in red. Centre: coronal brain slice at the level of the dotted red line of the cerebral view. Right: an enlargement of the amygdala showing its nuclei (Lateral, Basal, Central, Medial, ACC. Basal).

involved in processing representations and processes underlying reactions of fear, whether experienced personally or observed in others.

The cingulate gyrus

Mirror responses have also been found in the cingulate gyrus, which traditionally was subdivided into two main areas: area 24 rostrally and area 23 caudally (Brodmann, 1909). More recent parcellations distinguish four regions, distributed rostrocaudally: the anterior cingulate cortex (ACC), the median cingulate cortex (MCC), the posterior cingulate cortex (PCC), and the retrosplenial cingulate cortex (RSC), located behind the splenium of the corpus callosum. The ACC itself is composed of the subgenual anterior cingulate cortex (sACC),x and the pregenual anterior cingulate cortex (pACC) (Palomero-Gallagher et al., 2008, 2015). Similarly, MCC is composed of the anterior middle cingulate cortex (aMCC) and the posterior middle cingulate cortex (pMCC) (Vogt et al., 2003; Palomero-Gallagher et al., 2009).

From the functional point of view, the sACC is associated with the processing of negative events, while the pACC is involved in the decoding of positive events (Vogt, 2005). Both are linked with different portions of the amygdala. A large variety of functions have been attributed to MCC (feedback processing, encoding of the salience of the stimuli, association of rewards and actions, monitoring and motor control). However, a recent intracortical stimulation study by Fausto Caruana and colleagues at the University of Parma has shown that the function of this area is predominantly motor in nature (Caruana et al., 2018). Less clear is the function of the PCC, which seems to be involved in visual-spatial orientation, while very little is known yet about the RSCC.

At the end of the last century, William Duncan Hutchison and colleagues at the University of Toronto recorded the activity of single aMCC neurons. They found that a certain number of these neurons, located in the most posterior portion of the aMCC, responded to nociceptive stimuli. What was surprising was that some of these neurons also responded when the patients saw nociceptive stimuli being applied to the experimenter, demonstrating that these neurons have the mirror property (Hutchison et al., 1999). An fMRI study conducted by Tania Singer and colleagues at the University College London returned similar results; the posterior portion of their participants' aMCC became active when a nociceptive stimulus was applied to them but also when they were shown a video of electrodes being attached to the arm of a person dear to them, after having been told the electrodes would emit a painful shock. We will discuss how these data should be interpreted from a functional point of view in Chapter 3, but for the present suffice it to say that these data suggest that at least a part of the aMCC possesses the mirror property (Fig. 1.12).

However, the aMCC is not the only area of the cingulate gyrus to possess this property. Fausto Caruana and colleagues have run a series of studies stimulating the entire anterior portion of the cingulate gyrus from the pMCC to the pACC (Caruana et al., 2015). They discovered that the stimulation of the pACC could provoke a burst of laughter, accompanied by a feeling of hilarity. They also discovered, and this is particularly relevant to the purpose of this book, that the same portion of the pACC became active also when their subjects watched the sequence of a film during which an actor burst out laughing (Caruana et al., 2017).

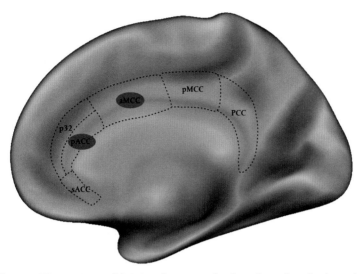

Fig. 1.12 The portions of the cingulate gyrus that have been found to have the mirror property, illustrated on a standard brain generated by Caret software.

Abbreviations: sACC = subgenual anterior cingulate cortex, pACC = pregenual anterior cingulate cortex, aMCC = anterior middle cingulate cortex, pMCC = posterior middle cingulate cortex, PCC = posterior cingulate cortex.

Mirror Neurons in other Species

So far we have been looking at mirror neurons in humans and non-human primates such as the macaque. In recent years, however, several studies have shown that the mirror property characterizes neurons in other animal species, even evolutionarily distant from each other. One such is that conducted by Wataru Suzuki and colleagues at the Riken Institute to investigate whether mirror neurons are present in the frontal cortex of the marmoset, a New-World monkey species that evolved separately from the Old-World species approximately 50 million years ago (Suzuki, Banno, Miyakawa et al., 2015). As the cortex of the marmoset is smooth and virtually without sulci (*corteccia lissencefalica*), Suzuki

31

and colleagues had first of all to record the activity of the superior temporal sulcus (STS) neurons, which, as in the macaque, discharge when actions are being observed (Suzuki, Tani, Banno et al., 2015). They then injected a luminescent retrograde tracer for an *in vivo* imaging technique by means of which they identified the areas in the ventrolateral frontal cortex from which to take their recordings. They used two experimental conditions: in the first, the marmoset observed another marmoset or the experimenter herself grasping an object such as a banana; in the second, the marmoset itself executed the action. The results revealed that the ventrolateral frontal cortex contained neurons that responded to grasping actions in both conditions, whether the animal was observing the actions being executed by others or executing them itself.

Mirror neurons have also been found in a nucleus (HVC) of the telencephalon of the forebrain of the swamp sparrow (*Melospiza georgiana*), a songbird with a distinctive monotone trill (Prather et al., 2008, see also Mooney, 2014). Kristi Prather and colleagues at Duke University focused their attention on this particular nucleus because it contains neurons that discharge while the bird is singing and others that fire when the bird itself is silent but another bird is singing nearby. In addition, from an anatomical point of view this nucleus is similar to the premotor cortex in primates. A number of its neurons project to the song motor nucleus RA, while another part innervates a striatal region of the basal ganglia (Area X) traditionally involved in perception and song learning.

While they were recording from the HVC, Prather and colleagues discovered that in addition to neurons with exclusively motor and auditory functions, there were others that fired in both conditions with a significant level of congruence, responding both while listening to a song sequence and while producing it. It is interesting to note that during the singing-related activity the pattern of discharge was not modulated by auditory feedback, to the extent that it did not change when this ceased, indicating that it is a motor response.

Moreover, a very recent study discovered mirror neurons in the motor cortex of rats (Viaro et al. 2021). Luciano Fadiga and colleagues at the University of Ferrara have provided evidence that about half of the recorded neurons discharged both while the rats were reaching for and grasping a food pellet and while they were observing another rat doing the same. It is interesting to note that none of the neurons seen to be responsive to observing the reaching-for and grasping actions responded while the rats were viewing another rat performing either a highly familiar action such as grooming or observing some graspable food alone. This suggests that mirror neuron responses may be highly selective in rats as well as in macaques and humans.

Finally, two recent studies have shown the presence of neurons with the mirror property in the hippocampus of rats (Danjo et al., 2018) and bats (Omer et al., 2018). It is now well known that the hippocampus and the entorhinal cortex play a key role in the construction of a dynamic representation of allocentric space, which is used for orientation purposes and for moving in surrounding space (Moser et al., 2008; Moser et al., 2017). Various types of neurons contribute to this representation, from place cells (O'Keefe & Nadel, 1978; Ulanovsky & Moss, 2007) to grid cells (Hafting et al., 2005) and boundary cells (Solstad et al., 2008), as well as those linked to head movements (Finkelstein et al., 2015). Shigeyoshi Fujisawa and colleagues at the Riken Institute wanted to ascertain whether place cells are able to represent the spatial position of others as well as that of self (Danjo et al., 2018), so they recorded the activity of single neurons from the CA1 area of the hippocampus of a rat while the animal was involved in the classic spatial T-maze orientation task. In order to receive a reward in this particular version of the task, the rat had to choose either the side opposite that occupied by another rat, or the same side. Their results showed that not only a significant part of the pyramidal CA1 cells represent the spatial position of both rats, but also that a subgroup of those cells exhibited identical receptive fields, responding both when the rat being recorded was in a certain place and when it saw the other rat in that same place.

Similarly, Nachum Ulanovsky and colleagues at the Weizmann Institute of Science of Rehovot recorded the activity of single neurons from the CA1 area of a bat's hippocampus. The bat had first to watch and then to imitate another bat flying through a tunnel in order to reach one of two balls positioned at its end (Omer et al., 2018). It was particularly interesting to see that while 70% of the recorded neurons behaved like typical place cells, representing the position of the bat during flight, the remaining 30% selectively responded to the position of the other bat flying through the tunnel, functioning as *social place cells*. Even more interestingly, approximately half of the social place cells also behaved as classical place cells, representing the position during the flight of both the observer bat and the bat being observed, which would mean that these neurons have the mirror property, or at least something very similar to it (Omer et al., 2018, p. 224).

The Chapter in Brief

These studies clearly show that neurons with the mirror property are to be found in many cerebral areas of a number of very different species, which would seem to indicate that this property reflects a fundamental functional principle of the nervous system, i.e. the same neurons and neural circuits can be used for processes and representations that concern both ourselves and others.

Another aspect, which is certainly not of secondary importance, has emerged from these studies; to the best of our knowledge at present, these processes and representations appear to underlie the most basic capabilities on which depends many of the possibilities we, and other species, have of successfully interacting with the environment. It is difficult to imagine a solution that would be evolutionarily more elegant and parsimonious than using the same processes and representations we recruit when executing actions or experiencing emotions ourselves, for observing them being executed or experienced by others.

This point will be discussed in depth in the final chapter of the book. Here we would like to start to reflect on what, if anything, is common to all the various mirror responses. From the earliest studies on the macaque and on humans, it has been hypothesized that the mirror responses are characterized by a transformation mechanism, known as the *mirror mechanism* (Rizzolatti et al., 2001; Rizzolatti & Sinigaglia, 2010).

To get a better idea of what this mechanism does, let us take another look at Fig. 1.2, which illustrates the behaviour of a typical F5 mirror neuron. As we have seen, area F5 is located in the ventral premotor cortex and modulates the spinal motoneurons both through connections with area F1 and the projections descending to the propriospinal system of the spinal cord (Borra et al., 2010).

The histogram in condition B shows the action potentials recorded by the neuron while the animal is grasping an object. Regardless of the aspect of the represented action, when that neuron fires it activates motor processes and representations that are similar to those that are triggered by the activation of F5 motor neurons. But what happens when the macaque observes the action of grasping rather than doing the grasping itself as in condition A? The *input* received from the neuron is different, of course. After all, the macaque is motionless in front of the experimenter. And what about the *output*? The output of the neuron in condition A has to be of the same kind that is recorded in condition B, as the information transmitted by the action potentials is the same in both cases. This suggests that the mirror response of the neuron in condition A entails a transformation of the incoming *sensory* representations into *motor* representations; more precisely into the same kind of *motor* representation that was recruited in condition B when the action was actually executed, not merely observed.

This is true not only for F5 mirror neurons, but for all the neurons with the mirror property encountered in this chapter. Certainly, it is one matter if the mirror response is recorded from the premotor cortex or even the primary motor cortex, quite another if it is recorded by centres such the insula or the amygdala. The incoming sensory representations, as well as the outgoing processes and representations, are very different. In spite of these differences, however, all mirror responses have the instantiation of a transformation mechanism in common, and this mechanism is always of the same kind.

In the following pages we will focus on the functioning of the mirror mechanism, starting with the domain of actions and progressing to that of the emotions, and finally to that of the so-called vitality forms that encompasses both. The choice of action as a starting point was by no means casual; the study of the mirror neurons in the action domain has provided the basis for interpreting the functioning of the mirror mechanism in other domains, starting from that of the emotions.

CHAPTER 2

ACTIONS

In the previous chapter, we have seen that brain areas with the mirror property are widespread in various species, humans included. In this chapter we will take a closer look at the parieto-frontal areas, which have been most frequently studied from a functional standpoint in both macaques and humans; in particular, we will try to clarify which processes and representations are involved in the mirror responses that occur while watching other people executing actions. Given the nature of the mirror mechanism, the starting point has to be the processes and representations involved in the planning and execution of these actions when we are executing them ourselves. After having identified which of the aspects of the actions we are observing can be represented by mirror neuron responses, we will discuss some recent studies suggesting that mirror responses can be modulated by the fact that the observed actions are executed in our surrounding space. Finally, we will show that these responses can also 'mirror' the action space of others, both when they are actually acting or simply have the possibility to do so.

Mirroring Brains. Giacomo Rizzolatti and Corrado Sinigaglia, Oxford University Press. © Oxford University Press 2023. DOI: 10.1093/oso/9780198871705.003.0002

Action Representation in the Macaque Brain

Goals and movements involved in executing an action

In Chapter 1 we have emphasized that the ethological approach was decisive for the discovery of some key functional properties that characterize most of the premotor neurons. Notably, extracellular recordings of single neurons have shown that the majority of the ventral premotor neurons (area F5) discharge selectively while specific actions are being executed (Rizzolatti et al., 1988). Some neurons discharged while a macaque was grasping a piece of food, others while the animal was holding an object in its hand, others again while it was engaged in cracking a nut, and so on. Those that discharged during grasping actions were found to respond selectively to a certain kind of grip, such as precision grip or whole-hand prehension. In addition, the temporal discharge profile varied from neuron to neuron; some fired at the end of the grasping action, a point which is characterized by a flexing of the fingers, others started firing when the hand was opening and continued to fire until the action was concluded, others again started firing even before the hand actually began to open, and in many cases only stopped when the nut finally cracked, i.e. when the action goal was achieved. So different were the characteristics of these F5 neurons that the presence of an 'action vocabulary' was hypothesized, whose main function was to facilitate the programming and control of the most common actions (Jeannerod et al., 1995; Rizzolatti et al., 2001).[1]

---

[1] With regard to grasping actions, some computational models have shown how the possibility of representing both the kind of grip and the timing that

One of the most interesting functional aspects to be discovered was that activation of F5 neurons depended on the macaque's action *goal*. We use the term *goal* to refer to the outcome(s) to which an action is directed, such as picking up a given object.[2] A natural question arises as to how it is possible to distinguish at *motor level* between the goal of an action and the *movements* that make the achievement of that goal possible. One way of doing this is to vary the goal while maintaining the movements constant, and vice versa.

Bend your index finger, for example, and think about what you can do by performing this simple movement; you can pick up a small object (precision grip) or grasp a larger object (whole-hand prehension). If a motor neuron responds differently during the execution of these two kinds of grip that require the index finger to be moved in a similar manner, it would be natural to conclude that this activation is not linked either to the muscles involved in the bending movement or to the movement's kinematic details. Fig. 2.1 shows an F5 neuron of this kind.

Of course, the fact that such neurons exist is not in itself enough to attribute the representation of possible action goals to F5 neurons.[3] This would require the existence of F5 motor neurons

characterized the various phases of the action significantly reduced the number of relevant parameters, greatly facilitating both the planning of the action and the controlling of its execution (Arbib et al., 1985; Mason et al., 2001; Santello et al., 2002; Tessitore et al., 2013).

[2] This is the everyday sense of the term in which we talk about the *goal* of someone's efforts. We will discuss this in depth in Chapter 6, showing that this minimal definition of action goal permits the introduction of conceptual distinctions that are useful when accounting for a process as complicated as the understanding of an action being executed by another person.

[3] It is true that bending a finger, or any other kind of muscle movement or contraction, could be considered as a possible action goal. There is no doubt about this. To put it simply, when we talk about possible action goals we are referring

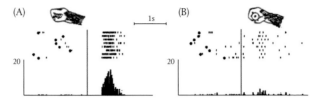

Fig. 2.1 An example of an F5 neuron responding (A) when the macaque bends a finger to grasp an object with a precision grip, but not when the animal bends it to grasp an object with a whole-hand prehension (B) (adapted from Gallese et al., 1996).

which would discharge when the goal remains the same, but the movements necessary to achieve it vary. Imagine grasping an object with your right hand, left hand, or mouth. The goal is the same but the movements are different, if only because different body parts are involved. If there were F5 motor neurons that discharged in a similar manner in all three conditions, it would be perfectly natural to assume that area F5 plays a key role in the motor representation of the goal(s) of an action.[4] Motor neurons of this kind have indeed been recorded in this area (see Fig. 2.2).

primarily to those outcomes that are typically attributed to the actions as goals, regardless of whether we are executing them ourselves or are observing someone else executing them. Usually we say that we grasp a glass or kick a ball, just as we usually think that the goal of the observed action is, for instance, to lift a book from the table. On the other hand, it is not surprising that action goals such as bending the index finger or extending the thumb can be represented motorically. What is more surprising is that action goals such as grasping, kicking, or lifting can be represented motorically. When we use the term 'possible action goals' in the following pages, we refer mainly to action goals of this kind.

[4] Throughout the book, when we speak about a motor representation of one or more possible action goals, we are referring to actions on a *small scale*, such as grasping, throwing, or moving an object but also walking, jumping, climbing, even playing a chord on a violin, or executing a dance step. In terms of means/goal relations, these are generally considered basic actions, whereas cooking pasta, going for a walk, executing one of Mozart's violin concertos or dancing as Clara

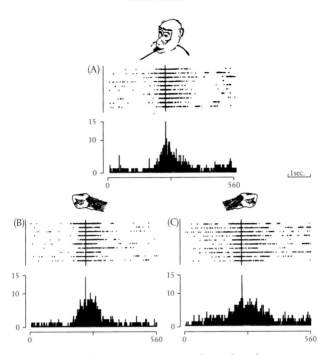

Fig. 2.2 An example of an F5 neuron responding when the macaque grasps a seed with its mouth (A), with the hand that is contralateral to the hemisphere in which the recorded neuron is located (B) and with the ipsilateral hand (C) (adapted from Rizzolatti et al., 1988).

Regarding the case illustrated in Fig. 2.2, it could be objected that the neuron's response does not represent grasping as a goal, but rather a motor synergy that in all three cases involves a mere open-and-close sequence. If we are to formulate a satisfactory reply to this objection, we will need to find a way to dissociate

in *The Nutcracker* are *medium- to large-scale actions*. Although discussing these latter actions is beyond the scope of this book, the possibility that one or more goals are represented motorically has a certain relevance also for medium to large scale actions, as every action that implies a form of movement includes a set of small-scale actions.

the grasping goal from the open-and-close motor synergy that is commonly used to attain it. How can this be achieved? Well, let's imagine picking up something, a sugar cube for example, with a pair of pliers. If you use a normal pair of pliers, the ones whose movements at the extremities replicate those of the hand, all you have to do to grasp the sugar cube is close your hand to close the instrument. However, let's assume that you only have a pair of the reverse pliers you normally use when extracting escargots from their shells, in which case the movements of the extremities are the reverse of your hand movements. In this case, to grasp the cube you have to close the pliers by opening your hand instead of closing it.

Some years ago, Alessandra Umiltà and colleagues at the University of Parma recorded the activity of F5 motor neurons while the macaque picked up food using both a pair of normal pliers and a pair of reverse pliers. They found that all the neurons that responded while the animal was using the regular pliers also responded when the reverse pliers were used. However, the most interesting discovery was that the discharge profile of these neurons was linked to the achievement of the goal (grasping the food), regardless of whether this required the animal to open or close its hand. In fact, as can be seen in Fig. 2.3, the neurons that fired when the macaque closed its hand to pick up the food with the regular pliers also fired when it opened its hand while using the reverse pliers to achieve the same goal.

In Chapter 1, we have drawn attention to the fact that the inferior parietal lobule is basically motor in nature and is somatotopically organized. Motor neurons with functional properties similar to F5 neurons have also been described in the PF and PFG areas, which are predominantly connected to mouth and hand movements

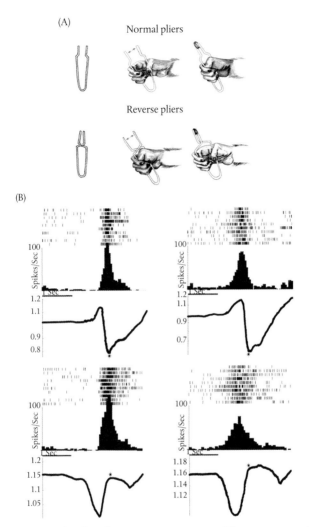

Fig. 2.3 An example of goal motor representation. The two types of pliers used are shown in (A). In order to pick up the food with the normal pliers, the macaque had to close its hand, but when using the reverse pliers it had to open it. The arrows indicate the direction of the movement of the extremities of the pliers. The graphs in (B) show the activity of two F5 neurons. The individual trials and the histograms indicate when the neuron fired while using the normal pliers (above) and the reverse pliers (below). The traces below each histogram indicate the position of the hand in that instant, recorded with the potentiometer and expressed as a function of the distance between the prongs of the pliers. When the trace descends, the hand is closing; when it is rising, the hand is opening and the distance between the prongs increases (adapted from Umiltà et al., 2008).

respectively. In fact, most of the neurons recorded in these areas represented the action goal to be executed, and not the individual movements necessary to achieve that goal (Rozzi et al., 2008). Similar results have been reported in the AIP area, which is located in the inferior parietal sulcus (Pani et al., 2014; Maeda et al., 2015).

One of the most interesting discoveries is the possibility that complex goals, hierarchically organized according to a typical means/goal instrumental relationship such as grasping food-to-lift-it-to-the-mouth, are also represented motorically just like individual goals (reaching for an object, grasping an object, lifting food to the mouth, etc.). Single neurons were recorded from the PFG while the macaque grasped a piece of food to put in its mouth or into a container (Fogassi et al., 2005). Approximately one-third of the recorded neurons fired in both conditions, so representing the goal of grasping as such. In contrast, during the reaching and grasping phase, two-thirds of the recorded neurons fired only if the grasping goal was an intermediate step to attaining a further goal, i.e. eating the piece of food or placing it in a container (Fig. 2.4).

It is worth noting that while in one of the early experiments the container was placed laterally with respect to the starting position of the macaque's hand, in a subsequent experiment it was placed on the animal's shoulder, not far from the mouth. This variant was necessary to ascertain that the effect did not depend on the direction of the movement of the hand following the grasping phase. The results showed that the PFG neurons that fired selectively when the macaque grasped the food to place it in the container in the proximity of its hand also fired when the container was placed close to the animal's mouth. On the contrary, the PFG neurons that fired when the macaque grasped the food in order to eat it, did not fire when the food was grasped with the goal of placing it in the

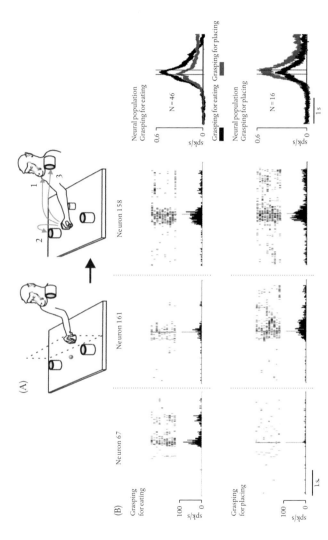

Fig. 2.4 Experimental paradigm. The container could be placed close to the hand or the mouth as the starting position. (B) Above: the activity of three IPL neurons while grasping in both conditions (grasping to eat, grasping to place). The red bars are aligned with the point in time when the macaque moved its hand from the starting position, while the green bars are aligned with the instant in which it touched the container. Below: responses of the population of neurons selective for grasping to eat and grasping to place. The two vertical lines in the two panels indicate, respectively, the instant in which the macaque touched the container and that in which it grasped it (adapted from Fogassi et al., 2005).

container, notwithstanding the fact that in both conditions the hand movement trajectory was very similar. Successively, Bonini et al. (2010) obtained analogous results with F5 neurons.

Goals and movements while observing action

So far we have discussed how frontal and parietal motor neurons discharge while an action is being executed. But what happens when the action is being *observed* instead of *executed*? In Chapter 1 we have seen that mirror neurons in the F5, PFG and AI areas fire both when we ourselves are acting and when we are observing someone else acting. The executed action and the observed action can be of the same kind: in this case, the mirror neurons are said to be *strictly congruent*. However, the two actions can be more or less similar in kind: in this case, the mirror neurons are considered as being *broadly congruent*. For example, sometimes a neuron that fires when the macaque grasps an object with a precision grip will also fire when the animal sees the experimenter or another macaque doing the same, or using a whole-hand prehension. It may also happen that a neuron that fires when a macaque grasps an object, fires also when the animal sees the experimenter or another macaque picking up or holding an object. Based on the various typologies, broadly congruent neurons represent approximately 70% of the total mirror neurons present in the macaque brain.

We have already seen that a fair number of the neurons of area F5 and the PFG and AIP areas that fire while an action is being executed, represent one or more possible goals. Is there evidence that this is true also for the mirror neurons in these areas when the action is being *observed* rather than *executed*? In other words, is there evidence that mirror responses reflect one or more possible action goals?

One way of assessing whether a mirror neuron represents a possible goal(s) while the execution of an action is being observed, is to work on the input, varying the sensory modality. Take cracking a peanut for example. If a mirror neuron fires when the animal is cracking a peanut, it is to be expected that this neuron would also fire when the animal *sees* or *hears* another individual cracking a peanut, as the action goal is the same in both cases. This was actually found by Evelyn Kohler and colleagues by recording F5 mirror neurons (Kohler et al., 2002). A percentage of the recorded neurons exhibited a similar discharge profile in four different conditions in which the macaque cracked open a peanut (action execution), watched and heard the experimenter cracking open a peanut (sight and hearing), watched the experimenter cracking open the peanut but with no accompanying sound (sight alone), and finally, heard the sound of the experimenter cracking the peanut but without seeing the action (hearing alone). The control experiments showed that non-specific factors such as arousal or emotional content related to the stimuli did not influence F5 neuron responses.

Another way of assessing the goal selectivity of mirror responses is to reduce the amount of sensory information available. Let's say you are watching a hand moving towards an apple, curling itself into the grasping position, ready to pick it up. Imagine that just before the hand reaches the apple, someone crosses your visual and you lose sight of the action for a split second. In spite of the fact that you do not actually see the conclusion of the action, the sight of the hand moving towards the apple would appear to be sufficient in itself to suggest that its goal, among all the various possibilities, is to grasp the fruit. If the mirror response can represent action goals, it is plausible that the mirror neurons which fire at the sight of a hand moving towards an object will discharge even if the information the brain receives regarding the end phase of the action is incomplete. Maria Alessandra Umiltà and colleagues recorded F5 neurons while a macaque was watching a grasping action from start to finish (complete visibility) and while the same animal was shown only the first part of the action (partial visibility) (Umiltà et al., 2001). In both conditions, the animal knew of the existence of an object at which the grasping action was directed. The results of this experiment confirmed that the neurons became active in both the full and partial visibility conditions.

Another way of studying mirror neuron goal selectivity is to keep the same goal but change the effector. Magali Rochat and colleagues (Rochat et al., 2010) recorded the activity of F5 mirror neurons while the animal picked up a piece of food with its hand or with a pair of reverse pliers, or watched these actions being executed. Almost all the neurons behaved as the neuron reported in Fig. 2.5, responding congruently both while observing the grasping action being executed manually and with reverse pliers, in spite of the fact that the goal was achieved using different effectors and with a different movement sequence.

We have already mentioned that a substantial portion of motor neurons in PFG and in area F5 are not only able to represent single goals such as grasping an object, but can also represent complex, hierarchically organized goals (grasping an object *to* lift it to the mouth or *to* put it in a container). The same paradigm used to study the activities of PFG and F5 neurons during the execution of a concatenation of actions characterized by an architecture of goals was

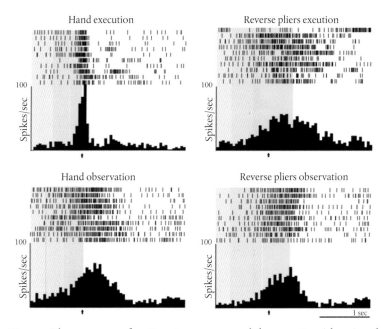

Fig. 2.5 The response of an F5 mirror neuron while executing (above) and observing (below) a grasping action with the hand (left) and a grasping action using reverse pliers (right). The coloured bands indicate four distinct phases: pink, the phase prior to the movement; purple, the opening phase of the grasping action; green, the closing phase of the grasping action; yellow, possession of the object (Rochat et al., 2010).

then used to investigate the responses of the mirror neurons of these areas while observing the same kind of actions.

In particular, while recording the activity of PFG mirror neurons when executing and observing grasping-by-hand actions, Luciano Fogassi and colleagues of the University of Parma discovered that a certain number of neurons discharged when observing a grasping-by-hand action regardless of its ulterior goal, but most of them fired selectively, depending on which action followed the first, thus achieving a composite goal of grasping *to* lift to the mouth or grasping *to* move to a container (Fogassi et al., 2005; Fig. 2.6).

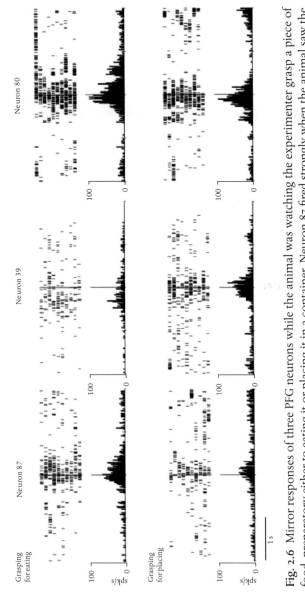

Fig. 2.6 Mirror responses of three PFG neurons while the animal was watching the experimenter grasp a piece of food, preparatory either to eating it or placing it in a container. Neuron 87 fired strongly when the animal saw the experimenter grasping the food to lift it to his mouth; the response became much weaker when, after having grasped the food, the experimenter placed it in a container. Neuron 39 did the opposite, while there were no substantial differences in the responses of Neuron 80 to the two conditions (adapted from Fogassi et al., 2005).

Using the same experimental paradigm, Luca Bonini and colleagues recorded the activity of F5 mirror neurons while their macaque watched the experimenter grasping a piece of food (or an object) to lift it to his mouth or place it in a container (Bonini et al., 2010). Two-thirds of the recorded neurons responded selectively while observing the grasping action, depending on whether the final goal was to lift the food to the mouth or place it in a container. The neuron discharge profile was not affected either by the position of the container or the type of object handled by the experimenter. Given the similarity of the mirror responses and the strong anatomical connections between areas F5 and PFG, it is natural to conclude that these two areas are at the base of a functional circuit linked to the representation of single and hierarchically organized goals during both execution and observation of grasping actions.

Action Representation in the Human Brain

Goals and movements

As has been done with the macaque, many studies with human participants have been dedicated to clarifying whether mirror responses are action goal selective, or whether they simply reflect the muscular pattern involved in the action or its kinematic profile. Although the techniques used with humans differed greatly with respect to those used with the macaques, the strategies were basically two. The first consisted in measuring if and how mirror responses change when the movements that are being observed vary, but the goals remain the same, and vice versa. The second consisted in investigating if and how mirror responses change according to the type of sensory information received, while the action goal remains the same.

Valeria Gazzola and colleagues adopted the first strategy a number of years ago in an fMRI experiment during which they showed fifteen volunteers a series of videos of actions executed by a human and a robotic arm and hand (Gazzola, Rizzolatti, Wicker et al., 2007). From a purely visual point of view, the human arm and hand were very different to the robotic version and the kinematic profiles of the actions observed, such as lifting a teabag out of a teacup, were clearly different when executed by the human arm and hand and by the robotic version. In spite of the very evident visual differences and regardless of which hand was used and the kinematics involved, the neuronal pattern activated by observing these actions was very similar to that which emerged when the actions were executed, with a clear overlapping of the frontal and parietal areas, in particular the premotor cortex and the inferior frontal gyrus, and the inferior parietal lobule respectively.

Two years later, Guy Orban and colleagues at the Catholic University of Lovanio carried out an fMRI study with human volunteers and specially trained macaques, using videos showing grasping actions executed by two hands, one human and one mechanical, as well as actions that involved the use of a candy, a ball, a rake, and pliers (Peeters et al., 2009). They discovered that regardless of whether the actions in the videos were executed by a human hand or a mechanical hand, with or without an instrument, a network of frontal parietal areas typically involved in actions with grasping goals was activated in both the human and macaque brains. Another discovery of no less importance was that observing actions executed with a tool activated a rostral portion of the inferior parietal lobule (and precisely, the anterior supramarginal gyrus) in the left hemisphere of the human brain, which is known to be selectively involved in producing tool actions. This did not occur in the macaque brain.

Luigi Cattaneo and colleagues of the University of Parma used normal and reverse pliers in a TMS experiment that provided even more convincing evidence that mirror responses can reflect the goal of an observed action, over and above the movements needed to attain it (Cattaneo et al., 2009). Stimulating the primary cortex and recording the motor-evoked potentials (MEPs) of the *opponens pollicis* muscle (the muscle involved in the movement of opposition to the thumb, typical of grasping), Luigi Cattaneo and colleagues found that observing a hand grasping with normal pliers caused an increase in the MEPs similar to that found when observing a hand grasping with reverse pliers, in spite of the fact that the movements of the thumb are completely different; grasping with normal pliers requires the thumb to bend, while grasping with reverse pliers requires it to extend. It was interesting to see that the MEP trend changed if the action being observed was a simple opening and closing of the pliers, without a specific goal. In this case, the MEPs only increased while watching the thumb bending, i.e. the movement that coincides with the closing of normal pliers and the opening of reverse pliers. This also occurred when their participants imagined grasping with both types of pliers, without actually executing the action; the MEPs increased in relation to the imaginary movement of the thumb, regardless of whether the movement would have closed normal pliers or opened the reverse type.

In these studies, the changes in the observed movements did not evoke a change in the mirror responses as the goal remained the same. The contrary, however, is also true; if the goal changes, the mirror responses should vary too, even if the movements are almost the same. Just to render the idea, imagine a mountaineer on a rock face reaching out to get an apple from his rucksack, and then imagine him reaching out to grip an outcrop. The hand movements in both cases may appear identical or very similar, but the goal itself is very different. Reasoning along these lines, Guy Orban and colleagues carried out an fMRI study to compare mirror responses while observing actions with different goals such as walking, climbing, or handling an object (Abdollahi et al., 2013). Not only did they find that different parietal-frontal circuits come into play when observing different actions, but they discovered that this also happened when, as in the example given above, the observed action is composed of movements that are very similar but their goals are different. Watching the hand of a mountaineer grasping an outcrop of rock does not activate the classic parieto-frontal circuit, but watching a hand picking up an object that can be manipulated does (Fig. 2.7).

Valeria Gazzola and colleagues adopted a variant to this strategy in a study involving two aplasic subjects born without arms and hands, who were asked to watch videos showing grasping-by-hand actions (Gazzola, van der Worp, Mulder et al., 2007). The same videos were watched by sixteen control subjects. They conducted a second experiment in which the aplasics were asked to pick up objects with their mouth or feet while the controls were instructed to pick up the objects with their hands as well. They found that while observing and executing the grasping actions both the aplasics and the controls activated a combination of parieto-frontal areas, of which a part had a clear, though different, somatotopy. In the aplasics, the areas activated while observing were, in part, those which were activated when they executed grasping actions with the mouth or foot, while in the case of the

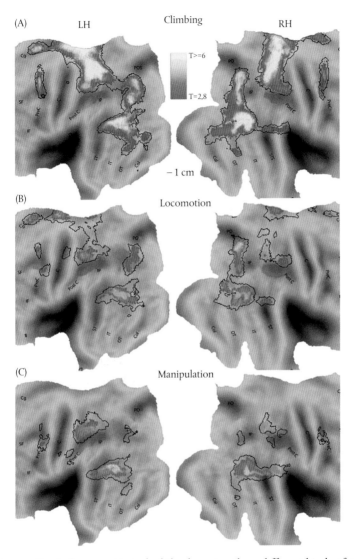

Fig. 2.7 Cortical areas activated while observing three different kinds of actions: (A) climbing, (B) locomotion, and (C) manipulation.

Abbreviations: Cg = cingulate sulcus, SFS = superior frontal sulcus, IFS = inferior frontal sulcus, PreCS = precentral sulcus, CS = central sulcus, PostCS = postcentral sulcus, IPS = intraparietal sulcus, POS = parieto-occipital sulcus, STS = superior temporal sulcus, ITS = inferior temporal sulcus, OTS = occipito-temporal sulcus, ColS = collateral sulcus (adapted from Abdollahi et al., 2013).

controls, they were, again in part, those which were activated while executing grasping-by-hand actions. The fact that a network endowed with the mirror property and involved in the production of grasping actions executed with the mouth or foot was activated in the two aplasics when they observed grasping actions executed by hand not only suggests that mirror responses are selective with respect to action goals, but also that this selectivity is not mandatorily constrained by the actual use of an effector (the hand, in this particular case), but depends rather on the possibility of representing and executing such action goals even with different parts of the body (mouth or foot, or hands).

With regard to the second strategy, which consists principally of scrutinizing mirror responses to changes in the kind of sensory information, James W. Lewis and colleagues at the West Virginia University carried out a fMRI study involving twenty subjects who were asked to listen to and then categorize two different kinds of sound, the first being associated with hand-manipulated tools while the second were animal sounds, mostly vocalizations (Lewis et al., 2005). By analysing the BOLD signal, they found that listening to the sounds of tools activated a network of mainly left-hemisphere parieto-frontal areas (including the premotor ventral cortex and the AIP, which are known to have the mirror property), while listening to animal sounds activated mainly the medial areas of the superior temporal gyrus.

Gazzola and colleagues obtained similar results from an fMRI study that aimed at identifying the areas which become active when actions performed with the hands or by mouth produce a particular sound (in the case of hand actions, the noise of paper being torn for example) and when listening to the sounds linked to those actions (Gazzola et al., 2006). The data indicate a clear overlapping in the activations of a parieto-frontal network, characterized by a strong somatotopy in the left premotor cortex. Indeed, a dorsal cluster of the left premotor cortex became active while executing hand actions and listening to the sounds associated with these actions, while a ventral cluster responded while executing mouth actions and listening to the sounds produced. It is worth noting that a fair part of the network also responded while observing these actions.

The discovery made by Emiliano Ricciardi and colleagues at the University of Pisa while conducting fMRI research with congenitally blind subjects is particularly interesting (Ricciardi et al., 2009). The authors asked the participants to listen to familiar sounds that are typically associated with certain actions (such as cutting a sheet of paper with a pair of scissors) and then to mime the action; they were also asked to listen to environmental sounds as a control condition. The congenitally blind subjects' performance was then compared with that of healthy sighted subjects, who were also required to watch a video of the actions producing the sounds they had listened to as well as a series of static environmental images. Listening to sounds associated with particular actions activated parieto-frontal areas in the congenitally blind group, in particular the ventral premotor cortex and the AIP area. This activation clearly overlapped both the response recorded during the motor pantomime in the congenitally blind subjects and the activation registered in the sighted subjects while listening to the same sounds and watching the videos of the actions with which the sounds are associated (Fig. 2.8). This indicates that not only did the sensitivity of the mirror responses to the action goals remain unvaried from one sensory modality to another, it was also independent of sight and was able to develop even in the absence of any visual experience whatsoever.

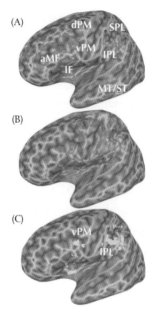

Fig. 2.8 Cerebral regions activated in congenitally blind subjects while (A) listening to sounds emitted by familiar actions, compared to listening to environmental sounds and (B) the motor pantomime of these actions compared to the rest condition. (C) shows the pattern of areas (the ventral premotor cortex and the AIP areas in particular) that were activated both by listening to sounds produced by familiar actions and by the miming of those actions (adapted from Ricciardi et al., 2009).

Abbreviations: aMF = anterior middle frontal cortex, IF = inferior frontal cortex, dPM = dorsal premotor cortex, vPM = ventral premotor cortex, IPL = inferior parietal lobule, SPL = superior parietal lobule, MT = middle temporal cortex, ST = superior temporal sulcus.

Goals and goal architecture

As in the macaque, mirror responses in humans can go beyond the representation of single goals; they can capture fairly complex architectures, generally structured as instrumental relations in which the achievement of one goal represents the means to achieve another. Marco Iacoboni with a group of researchers at the

University of California of Los Angeles (Iacoboni et al., 2005) carried out an fMRI experiment in which they showed their participants three sets of movie clips: the first set presented a number of objects (a teapot, a mug, a glass, a plate, etc.) that suggested two different situations (before and after drinking a mug of tea); the second set showed only a hand grasping a mug with a precision grip or whole-hand prehension, while in the third set the same hand was shown grasping the mug in the tea-drinking context, with the two grips mentioned above, suggesting either that the mug was being lifted for the purpose of drinking or to move it from the table. Comparing the cerebral activations induced by observing the three sets of images, the authors found that when the participants saw the hand grasping the mug in a situation that clearly implied the purpose of lifting it either to drink or to move it away, there was a significant increase in the activity in the dorsal portion of the posterior section of the inferior right frontal gyrus, which, as we have seen, is a fundamental node of the network of parieto-frontal areas endowed with the mirror property.

Using similar stimuli in a high-density EEG study integrated with neuroimaging, Stephanie Ortigue and colleagues at the University of California of Santa Barbara investigated the temporal dynamics of the cerebral areas involved in encoding the goals of observed actions (Ortigue et al., 2010). These authors found that a pattern of cortical activity characterized by four distinct temporal phases resulted when their participants observed a hand holding a mug with a grasp and in a situation that implied that the final goal was to lift it to drink from it or to clear it away. The first phase was characterized by bilateral posterior cortical activations and the second by strong activation of the left posterior temporal and inferior parietal cortices as well as by a remarkable decrease of activation in the right hemisphere; the third phase was characterized by a significant increase of the activations of the right temporo-parietal region, while the final phase saw a significant global decrease of cortical activity accompanied by the appearance of activation of the orbito-frontal cortex. The authors hypothesized that the strong activation of the left hemisphere was linked to the representation of a single goal (e.g. grasping the mug), while the successive activation of the right hemisphere reflected the representation of the entire architecture of which the goal was part (grasping the mug *in order to* drink from it or *in order to* move it).

An elegant study by Luigi Cattaneo and colleagues at the University of Parma in 2007 contributed significantly to supporting the hypothesis that mirror responses in humans can be modulated by the final goal of the observed action, as happens in macaques (Cattaneo et al., 2007). The authors took electromyographic recordings of the mouth-opening mylohyoid (MH) muscle while their participants were engaged in two types of tasks, one executing an action and the other watching an action being executed (Fig. 2.9A). In the first task, the participants were instructed either to take a piece of food and lift it to their mouths or to take a piece of paper and place it in a container located on their shoulders, while in the second task they were asked to watch the experimenter executing the same kind of action. A strong increase in the electromyographic activity of the MH muscle was recorded both when the participants picked up the food to put it in their mouths and when they observed the experimenter doing so. Moreover, in both conditions this increase was already evident during the reaching phase, i.e. when the participants' and the experimenter's hands started to move towards the piece of food (Fig. 2.9B), while there was no activation of the MH muscle when the participants moved the piece of

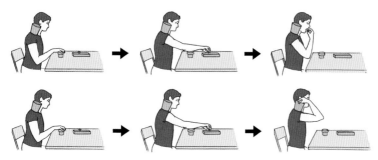

Fig. 2.9A Schematic representation of the tasks of Experiments 1 and 2. (Top) The individual reaches for a piece of food located on a touch-sensitive plate, grasps it, lifts it to the mouth, and finally eats it. (Bottom) The individual reaches for a piece of a paper located on the same plate, grasps it, and puts into a container placed on their shoulder.

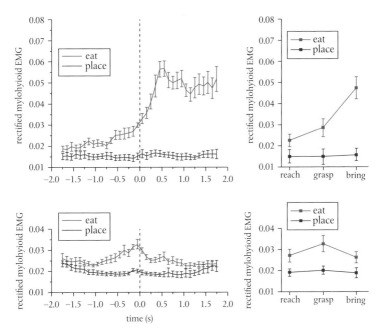

Fig. 2.9B Time course of the EMG activity of the MH muscle when the participants executed the action themselves (above) and observed it being executed (below). The lifting-to-the-mouth action is indicated in red and the placing-the-paper action in blue. (Right) The dashed vertical line indicates the instant when the hand starts to lift the object (adapted from Cattaneo et al., 2007).

paper or observed the experimenter moving it. The pattern of electromyographic activation indicated that the final action goal could be represented motorically from its initial phases, both while an action is being executed and when it is being observed.

Mirroring Actions

Taken together, the studies we have mentioned above support the existence of neurons in the premotor cortex and inferior parietal lobule that are able to represent one or more possible goals, both when we ourselves execute an action and when we watch someone else executing it. These neurons have a specific synaptic connection pattern; whether they are activated while an action is being executed or being observed, this pattern remains the same, as does the content of what they represent.

Consider the mirror neurons of the F5 or PFG/AIP areas, for example; these neurons respond to a specific action goal such as grasping, both when we ourselves execute a grasping action and when we observe it being executed by another person. As anticipated in Chapter 1 (pp. 35–36), the response of these neurons involves the transformation of the incoming representations into *motor* representations regarding that specific action goal. Of course, when we are executing the action ourselves the incoming representations are different to when we are watching someone else executing it; the former are *motor or motor-like* representations that originate in the areas of the prefrontal cortex while the latter are *visual* or *sensory* representations that usually originate in the temporal lobe. However, the outgoing representation, i.e. the *motor* representation of a goal such as grasping, does not change.

When this representation is recruited while an action is being observed, it inevitably triggers the same kind of processes and representations as when it is recruited during the execution of the action. This means, among other things, that the responses of the mirror neurons in area F5 or the PFG/AIP areas involve a transformation of the sensory representations induced by observing an action into the motor representations of one or more possible goals—representations that in no way differ from those that we would recruit if, rather than observing the action, we were to execute it ourselves. Due to this transformation, the sensory information regarding the observed action is therefore processed by those same motor centres that are activated when the action is executed in the first person (Fig. 2.10).[5]

In this regard, we know that area F5, and F5p in particular, modulates motoneurons as it projects directly both to area F1 and to the propriospinal system of the spinal cord (Borra et al.,

---

[5] Karl Friston, James Kilner, and Chris Firth have delineated an alternative interpretation of the mirror mechanism in the framework of what is known in literature as *predictive coding*, that is not incompatible with what we have presented here (Kilner et al., 2007, see also Friston et al., 2011). Briefly, predictive coding consists in predicting sensory effects starting from their cause, and is based on 'a minimization of prediction error though recurrent or reciprocal interactions among levels of a cortical hierarchy'. In the case of the mirror mechanism, given the functional and anatomical connections between the various areas endowed with the mirror property, the idea is that 'the prediction error encoding higher-level attributes will be expressed as evoked responses in higher cortical levels of the mirror neuron systems. For action observation the essence of this approach is that, given a prior expectation about the goal of the person we are observing, we can predict their motor commands. Given their motor commands we can predict the kinematics on the basis of our own action system. The comparison of this predicted kinematics with the observed kinematics generates a prediction error. This prediction error is used to update our representation of the person's motor commands. Similarly, the inferred goals are updated by minimizing the prediction error between the predicted and inferred motor commands' (Kilner et al., 2007, p. 161). While appreciating the predictive coding approach, we do entertain certain perplexities regarding the assumption that the sensorimotor transformations

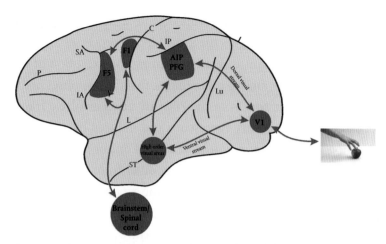

Fig. 2.10 The principal anatomical, cortical, and descending pathways by which sensory representations regarding observed actions are transformed into motor representations of possible action goals that are normally recruited when the actions are executed rather than being observed by others.

Abbreviations: IA = inferior arcuate sulcus, C = central sulcus, IP = intraparietal sulcus, AIP = anterior intraparietal area, L = lateral fissure, Lu = lunate sulcus, P = principal sulcus, V1 = primary visual area, SA = superior arcuate sulcus, ST = superior emporal sulcus.

2010). We also know that area F5 and the PFG and AIP areas are strongly interconnected, and that the PFG and AIP areas are in turn connected to the higher-order visual areas of the STS (Rozzi et al., 2006). Comparing the functional characteristics of the STS neurons allows us to further clarify the nature of the sensorimotor

induced by mirror responses would have the function of minimizing the prediction error merely at the kinematic level, whereas the *a priori* expectations regarding the observed action goals would be generated externally to the motor areas endowed with the mirror property (Kilner, 2011). Although the mirror mechanism can be modulated top-down, the data we have reported in the previous sections indicate that the mirror responses of the parieto-frontal areas can represent possible action goals, going beyond the purely kinematic features of the observed action. This will be dealt with in greater detail in Chapters 5 and 6, distinguishing between the different levels at which action goals can be represented.

transformations induced by the mirror neuron activity in area F5 and the PFG/AIP area while observing actions being executed.

It is well-known that there are neurons in the STS that respond to complex visual stimuli, as for example the sight of a hand grasping an object (Perrett et al., 1985, 1989). However, the fact that these STS neurons respond while observing grasping actions does not mean that they represent the observed action in the same way that F5 and PFG/AIP mirror neurons do. The studies cited in the preceding pages clearly indicate that the neurons in these areas may represent one or more action goals with various degrees of generality. As we have mentioned earlier, there are F5 and PFG/AIP mirror neurons that do not modify their discharge profile when the action is executed with different effectors (hand, mouth, etc.) or even with tools (pliers and reverse pliers, for example) that require opposite movement sequences. There are F5 and PFG/AIP mirror neurons that activate while observing an action with a particular goal, but not when the goal appears to be different, even if its kinematic profile is very similar. There is no evidence to date that STS neurons encode action goals, going beyond the representation of specific, even complex, visual action features, as F5 and PFG/AIP mirror neurons do. In fact, to the best of our knowledge, the only study that was conducted with the precise objective of evaluating how the parieto-frontal regions endowed with the mirror property and the visual areas of STS contribute to the representation of action, would appear to indicate the contrary.

In this study, Luigi Cattaneo and colleagues at the University of Trento used the TMS technique with an adaptation paradigm (Cattaneo et al., 2010). On the basis of this paradigm, repeated exposure to a visual stimulus results in a decrease in the response of the neurons involved in the representation of that stimulus, which at behavioural level results in longer reaction times. If TMS is applied to the areas that are thought to be involved in the representation of the 'adaptive' stimulus just before it is shown to the participant, it induces a change of state in these areas that restores the intensity of the pre-adaptation response. At a behavioural level, this translates into a shortening of the reaction times compared to those recorded in the phase following the adaptation.

In this particular study, the visual stimuli that were to induce the adaptation were videoclips showing two actions (grasping and pushing), executed by two different effectors (hand and foot) and related to two different target objects (a ball and a cube). The participants were instructed to respond as quickly as possible to an image representing a hand or a foot grasping or pushing a ball or a cube, and to indicate whether the action observed in the image was the same or different to the action seen in the adaptive stimulus. TMS pulses were applied to three distinct cortical regions—the ventral premotor cortex, the inferior parietal lobe, and the STS—just before the presentation of the test images. When TMS was applied to the ventral premotor cortex and the inferior parietal lobe, there was an evident shortening of reaction times to the adapted actions when the goal of the observed action was of the same kind (grasping or pushing), independently of the effector used. When TMS was applied to STS, however, this shortening of the reaction times to the adapted actions occurred only when the effector involved was the same. This indicates that, while action representation in the premotor and inferior parietal cortices regarded the action goal and not the specific means of achieving it, in the STS it remained anchored to the effector type.

Although no systematic study has yet been made at single neuron level of the differences in action representation between F5 and PFG/AIP mirror responses and the purely visual responses of the STS, it seems unlikely that STS neurons could represent observed actions with the same degree of generality shown by F5 and PFG/AIP neurons. Let's say that an STS neuron responds selectively to the sight of a hand grasping something, specifically representing the visual aspects that enable the identification of a hand in movement with a particular grip; now, the question is how could that same neuron also respond selectively to the sight of a mouth executing the same kind action, given that from the visual point of view the stimuli are very different. One solution to this could be to call on an associative process, adopting a strategy similar to that used by Yasushi Miyashita and colleagues to explain the neuronal coding of the long-term visual memory in the temporal lobe (Miyashita, 1988; Sakay & Miyashita, 1991). However, association in STS would necessarily involve multiple visual aspects of temporally and spatially contiguous body parts in movement, and it is unlikely that it would be able to capture the observed action goal when it is achieved by means of a different effector or even a tool. F5 and PFG/AIP mirror neurons on the other hand are able to represent not only a single action goal such as grasping achieved with any effector or tool, but also an architecture of goals hierarchically organized on a means/goal basis, e.g. grasping-*to*-lift-to-the-mouth or grasping-*to*-move (Fogassi et al., 2005; Bonini et al., 2010). This makes figuring out how STS neurons could do the same by processing purely visual aspects of action very challenging indeed.

Action goal representation of F5 and PFG/AIP mirror neurons differs from that of STS neurons because of its *motor* format. This kind of representation is typically recruited in action execution and its primary function is to facilitate motor preparation and control. When a representation of this kind is recruited while observing an action, its content and format are the same as in motor preparation and control. This explains why this kind of representation is neither linked to a specific visual aspect of the observed action nor to a single sensory modality. It also explains why mirror responses depend mainly on how action goals are represented motorically, as has been demonstrated by the numerous experiments carried out with people endowed with specific motor skills.

One such is the fMRI experiment run some years ago by Beatriz Calvo-Merino and colleagues, who demonstrated that the mirror responses to the observation of various kinds of action varied in function of the observer's level of expertise in those kinds of actions (Calvo-Merino et al., 2005). Their participants were divided into three groups: dancers expert in classical ballet, martial arts teachers expert in capoeira and absolute beginners who had never set foot on a dance floor. When a video of capoeira steps was shown to the groups, the parieto-frontal areas endowed with the mirror property became active in the capoeira teachers to a far greater extent than in the other two groups. As was to be expected, the video showing classical ballet steps evoked a greater mirror response in the ballet dancers than in the capoeira teachers or the beginners.

Further experiments have been done with pianists. Bernhard Haslinger and colleagues at the Technical University of Munich compared the cerebral activity of expert pianists and musically naïve controls while they watched fingers playing some chords or simply serial finger-thumb opposition movements with or without synchronous piano sound (Haslinger et al., 2005).

The results showed greater activation of the pianists' parieto-frontal mirror areas, but only when watching the movement of the fingers playing the chords. It is interesting to note that these movements, but only these, also recruited auditory areas in the pianists. Similarly, Martin Lotze and colleagues at the University of Tübingen conducted a TMS study to measure the primary motor cortex activity in pianists listening to a piece of music before and after rehearsing it (D'Ausilio et al., 2006). After the pianists had rehearsed the piece, the authors noted a significant increase in the level of excitability of the primary motor cortex. Interestingly, it took only thirty minutes of practising to reach such a motor facilitation effect, although it took much longer (approximately 5 days) to achieve a more lasting effect. Subsequent studies (Candidi et al., 2014 using TMS and Panasiti et al., 2016 using EEG) found that when skilled pianists (as opposed to expert musicians who do not play the piano and beginners) passively observed a sequence of chords being played by another person, not only was a degree of cerebral activity evoked that was very similar to that when they actually played the chords themselves, but the manner in which they processed the errors they noted in the other person's execution of the chords was very similar to that with which they processed their own.

Of course, given the factorial design of these studies, it could be objected that at the most they indicate that expertise can modulate mirror responses; they do not provide evidence that this modulation depends primarily on the capacity to motorically represent possible action goals. Those who become skilled pianists and dancers have not only acquired the capacity to motorically represent particular chords and dance steps, but they have also developed the capacity to represent them visually, because they are continuously exposed to these actions, observing them as they are executed by their maestro, dance teacher, or partner.

To tackle this issue, Beatriz Calvo-Merino and colleagues conducted another study with the aim of measuring the contribution of motor and visual expertise to mirror responses. To do this they compared two groups of participants with different levels of motor competence but similar visual expertise with regard to the actions to be observed (Calvo-Merino et al., 2006). There are steps in ballet that are traditionally executed by danseurs and others by ballerinas, and steps that both can execute; both have visual expertise in all the dance steps, but their motor expertise is limited to the steps they themselves perform. But what happens in the brain of a ballet dancer who is shown a video of dance steps in which they are motorically expert and which belong to their motor repertoire, and other steps, belonging to the repertoire of other dancers, of which their experience is only visual? Beatriz Calvo-Merino's results clearly indicate that *motor* expertise has a greater impact on the activation of the areas endowed with the mirror property, and specifically on the left premotor cortex and the bilateral intraparietal sulcus. The activation in these areas, in fact, was greatest when the dancers were watching the steps they were expert in, compared to when they were observing those which did not belong to their motor repertoire.

Similar results were obtained by Emily Cross and colleagues from an fMRI study in which expert dancers were asked to learn and rehearse novel, complex, whole-body dance sequences five hours a week for five weeks (Cross et al., 2006). Each week the dancers were scanned and their cerebral activity measured while they watched or imagined executing both the dance steps they had learned and others they had not yet practised. At the end of each session they were asked to respond to a questionnaire that measured the level of competence they thought they had reached that week. On comparing the data from the observation and imagination of the steps learned and the observation and imagination of the steps still to be learned, the researchers found that the activation of the premotor and inferior parietal areas endowed with the mirror property was much stronger in the steps-learned condition. Even more interesting was their finding that the activity of the mirror areas correlated both with the level of motor expertise acquired when the dancers were scanned and the level of competence in the steps that they considered they had mastered from one week to the next.

A Space for Action

So what have we seen so far? On the one hand, we have seen that mirror neuron responses involve a transformation of the *sensory* representations induced by the observation of an action into the *motor* representations of one or more possible goals similar to those that would be recruited if the observer were to execute that kind of action. On the other hand, we have seen that mirror responses depend primarily on the capacity to represent possible action goals motorically. The greater this capacity, the greater will be the possibility of mirroring these goals when actions are observed rather than being executed, as is borne out by the recent studies on the role of motor expertise in observing action.

A large number of studies over the last few years have convincingly shown that mirror responses can be modulated by the fact that actions we observe fall within our own peripersonal space. *Peripersonal* space is usually defined as the space surrounding an organism, encompassing everything that can be reached without using any form of locomotion. Peripersonal space differs from *personal* (or cutaneous) space that corresponds to the organism's bodily surface and also from *extrapersonal* space that includes everything which is not within immediate reach (Rizzolatti et al., 1997).

Peripersonal space is known to be represented by a network of parieto-frontal areas whose main nodes have been identified in the macaque brain in the dorsal portion of the ventral premotor cortex (area F4) and in the ventral intraparietal area (VIP) (Fogassi et al., 1992; Colby et al., 1993). F4 neurons fire when movements are made with the goal of reaching an object (with the hand) (Gentilucci et al., 1988) or avoiding something (with the head or the rest of the body) (Graziano, 2018). Some of these motor neurons also respond to somatosensory stimuli (unimodal neurons), while others respond to both somatosensory and visual stimuli (bimodal neurons; Gentilucci et al., 1988; Fogassi et al., 1992, 1996; Graziano et al., 1994; see Fig. 2.11). Finally, there are other neurons that respond to somatosensory, visual, and auditory stimuli (trimodal neurons), but these are relatively rare (Graziano et al., 1999). Bimodal neurons have also been detected in the VIP area (Colby et al., 1993; Duhamel et al., 1998). fMRI experiments have shown that there is a similar homologous parieto-frontal circuit in humans (Filimon et al., 2007).

Peripersonal space is also known to be a *space for action*. Not only is it encoded in somatic coordinates and represented in terms of

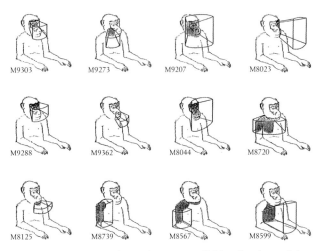

Fig. 2.11 Somatosensory and visual receptive fields of F4 bimodal neurons. The shaded areas indicate the somatosensory receptive fields; the solid shapes drawn around the body parts of the macaque delineate the visual receptive fields, which are anchored to the corresponding somatosensory receptive fields and are of various shapes and size, with a depth ranging from a few centimetres to 40–50 cm (adapted from Fogassi et al., 1996).

potential action goals (reaching, avoiding), its boundaries embrace everything that is within the range of action.[6] If the range of the action changes, so does the range of the peripersonal space, as Atsushi Iriki and colleagues so brilliantly demonstrated with an experiment involving tool use by macaques (Iriki et al., 1996). Recording single cells from the caudal postcentral gyrus they discovered that the visual receptive fields of the bimodal neurons expanded when the macaque used a rake to reach and retrieve pieces of food that would otherwise have been inaccessible. They also found that if the animal stopped using the rake but continued to

---

[6] The notion of peripersonal space and its nature as space for action is discussed in greater depth in Chapter 3 of our previous book (Rizzolatti & Sinigaglia, 2008).

hold it, the receptive fields returned to their normal extension (see also Ishibashi et al., 2000). Similar results have been obtained in experiments with brain-damaged patients suffering from visual tactile extinction[7] or spatial hemineglect[8] and with healthy subjects.[9]

Given the nature of peripersonal space, Vittorio Caggiano and colleagues wondered whether the mirror neuron response could be modulated by the fact that the observed action was either within or out of the observer's reach (Caggiano et al., 2009). They devised an experimental paradigm recording F5 mirror neurons, in which

[7] It is known that patients affected by visual tactile extinction tend not to notice the presence of a tactile stimulus on the contralesional hand if a visual distractor is concurrently placed close to the other hand. This effect usually disappears when the distractor is out of the ipsilesional hand's reach. That said, it has been shown that if the patient is actively using a rake, the visual tactile extinction occurs also when the distractor is out of the hand's reach, but not of that of the tool (Farnè & Làdavas, 2000; Maravita et al., 2001; Farnè et al., 2005).

[8] Patients with spatial hemineglect, caused mainly by damage to the right parietal lobe, generally have no awareness of stimuli present in the contralesional hemispace. Some may have selective spatial hemineglect for peripersonal and extrapersonal space. Various studies have shown that the performance of patients with this type of disorder can deteriorate (or improve) in a classic bisection task if executed with a rod rather than a laser pointer as the former enables the patient to physically reach the line to be bisected, while the latter 'delegates' the action to the laser dot at a distance (Berti & Frassinetti, 2000; Pegna et al., 2001; Ackroyd et al., 2002; Neppi-Mòdona et al., 2007). More recently a number of studies have shown that extrapersonal space can be remapped as peripersonal space not only by bisecting a line but also by observing it being bisected by another person (on the condition that the observer is actually able to execute the task) (Costantini, Frassinetti, Maini et al., 2014).

[9] In a study conducted some years ago, Marcello Costantini et al. showed that using a pair of pliers to reach and grip objects that would otherwise be out of reach and watching someone else executing the same action (as long as the person observing the action was in fact able to physically execute it themselves), resulted in an extension of the observer's peripersonal space for the duration of the task (Costantini et al., 2011). It is interesting to note that if instead of using a tool to reach a distant object, you walk towards it, your peripersonal space 'walks' with you (Berti et al., 2002).

a macaque watched the experimenter grasping objects inside and outside its peripersonal space. The results showed that in approximately 50% of the mirror neurons recorded, the response returned was different, depending on whether the action the animal was watching occurred inside or outside its peripersonal space: 25% of the neurons responded preferentially to actions executed within its peripersonal space and the other 25% to those executed outside its peripersonal space (Fig. 2.12).

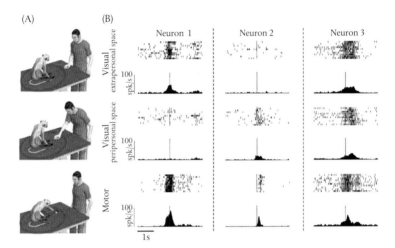

Fig. 2.12 Mirror neuron responses while a macaque watched actions being executed in its peripersonal and extrapersonal space. (A) Schematic view of the experimental paradigm. The circle around the animal's body delimits the reaching distance range (peripersonal space). The monkey observes the experimenter grasping an object in its extrapersonal space (left) and peripersonal space (centre). The monkey grasps an object in front of it, in its peripersonal space (right). (B) Responses of three mirror neurons in the three experimental conditions illustrated in (A). Neuron 1 responds selectively when watching the action in the extrapersonal space, while neuron 2 responds when watching the action in the peripersonal space. Neuron 3 did not show any spatial modulation. All three neurons discharged while the action was being executed (adapted from Caggiano et al., 2009).

Strikingly, the mirror responses did not reflect the physical distance between the animal and the action it was observing. When a transparent barrier was placed between the experimenter and the animal while the former was executing a grasping action at the same distance that usually evoked a mirror response in the original condition, the mirror neurons that were selective for peripersonal space ceased firing, as if the placing of the barrier caused that portion of space originally mapped as peripersonal space to become extrapersonal space. Vice versa, before the barrier was placed, the neurons selective for extrapersonal space were silent but when the barrier was introduced, they started firing.

Similar results were obtained in a more recent study by Luca Bonini and colleagues who trained macaques to execute a task requiring the animal to watch an object and grasp it at a given signal or observe the experimenter executing the same kind of action (Bonini et al., 2014). The observed action was executed by the experimenter within the animal's peripersonal or extrapersonal space. At the beginning of each observation trial the macaque not only saw the object, but also the experimenter's hand, motionless, close to it. As in the experiment conducted by Vittorio Caggiano and colleagues in 2009, part of the F5 mirror neurons responded selectively when the action was executed in the macaque's peripersonal space, while another part responded when the action was executed in its extrapersonal space; there were also a good number that responded in both conditions.

In the same study Luca Bonini and colleagues also recorded F5 canonical and canonical-mirror neurons. As we have seen in Chapter 1 (p. 4), canonical neurons associate visual to motor responses, selectively discharging both when objects with different shapes and sizes were actually grasped and also when they were merely viewed. Canonical-mirror neurons combine mirror and canonical properties by not only responding while an action is being directed at an object with a specific shape and size, but also while this kind of action is being executed by other people, and even simply at the sight of an object with that particular shape and size. Practically all of the canonical neurons recorded fired only when the object appeared in the animal's peripersonal space. Regarding canonical-mirror neurons, while the mirror responses were uniformly distributed between peripersonal and extrapersonal space, approximately 70% of the cases of canonical responses were linked to peripersonal space (Fig. 2.13). The authors found that the remaining 30% of the canonical-mirror neurons responded even when the object was placed out of the animal's reach but close to the experimenter's hand, almost as if it represented the target of a potential action, regardless of the agent.

Similar results have been obtained in studies carried out with human subjects. Marcello Costantini and colleagues conducted an experiment in which the participants were asked to mimic the action of grasping with the right or left hand as soon as a go-signal came into view (Costantini et al., 2010; see also Cardellicchio et al., 2011). The go-signal consisted of the image of a mug with its handle aligned (or unaligned) with the hand to be moved. Although the information about the position and the orientation of the mug was irrelevant for the mimicking task, when the handle of the mug was congruent with the hand to be moved the participants tended to be quicker in mimicking the

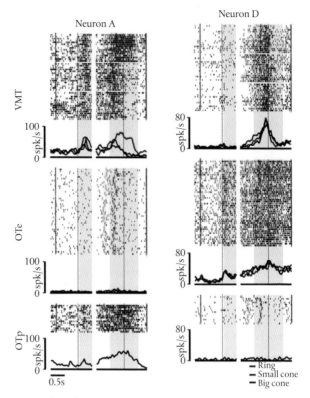

Fig. 2.13 Examples of two canonical-mirror neurons. The top panels show the responses of the neurons during the visuomotor executive task (VMT), those in the centre during the observation task, when the object and the action being observed were in the animal's extrapersonal space (OTe). The bottom panels show the responses of the neurons during the observation task when the object and the action were located outside its peripersonal space (OTp). Note the different selectivity with respect to the observation of objects and actions in the peripersonal and extrapersonal space (adapted from Bonini et al., 2014).

grasping action (see also Tucker & Ellis, 1998). This effect, known as the spatial alignment effect (Bub & Masson, 2010), was present only if the mug seemed to be in the participants' peripersonal space. If the mug appeared to be outside the participants' reach or was placed behind a transparent barrier so as to appear ungraspable, the participants took the same time to start mimicking the grasping action as when the presented mug was both congruent and incongruent with the hand to be moved. Even more interestingly, if the mug appeared to be far from the participants but close to a potential agent such as an avatar, the spatial alignment effect reappeared, but only if there was no transparent barrier between the avatar and the mug (Costantini et al., 2011; see also Cardellicchio et al., 2013).[10]

Akira Murata and colleagues made an exceptionally interesting discovery some years ago when studying mirror neurons in the macaque (Ishida et al., 2010). Their findings showed that the mirror response does not stop at the observed action and can even reflect the peripersonal space of another individual. While recording single cells from the VIP area, the authors found bimodal neurons that responded to visual stimuli not only in the macaque's peripersonal space but also in that of the experimenter who was standing at a distance from the animal, face on. The visual stimuli were presented to the macaque at a distance that was gradually modified, either shortened from 120 cm to 10 cm or extended from 10 cm to 120 cm, after which an experimenter sat on a chair in front of the animal at a distance of 120 cm, and passed his hand or a stick in front of his own face or other body parts. Many of the bimodal neurons recorded from the VIP area showed receptive visual fields connected to receptive tactile fields and anchored to a specific body part of the macaque (face, trunk, forearm, hand, leg,

---

[10] Similar results have been obtained in an experiment with congenitally blind participants (Ricciardi et al., 2017). These findings are significant as they show that representation of peripersonal space can be developed independently of visual experience.

etc.). The neurons discharged selectively when a visual stimulus appeared in the macaque's peripersonal space, in the proximity of the corresponding body part. No activity was recorded when the stimulus appeared at 120 cm from the animal. This changed, however, when the experimenter stood in front of the animal at this distance. Indeed, a significant portion of the VIP bimodal neurons fired as long as the stimulus was close to the experimenter's corresponding body part (Fig. 2.14). When he moved away, the neurons stopped firing. It is interesting to note that the responses of the VIP bimodal neurons were stronger when the stimulus appeared at a distance of 30 cm from either the macaque or the experimenter, suggesting that these neurons may represent our own peripersonal space and that of others.

Akira Murata and colleagues did not extend their research to investigate whether these VIP neurons had motor properties. However, as we have mentioned before, the VIP area is closely connected to area F4 where peripersonal space is motorically represented in terms of possible action goals (to reach for or to avoid). Therefore, we can hypothesize that the visual responses of VIP neurons evoke motor representations of potential actions directed either at objects within reach or at specific parts of the body (Rizzolatti & Sinigaglia, 2015). It must be emphasized that this is indeed a hypothesis, and though anatomically and functionally plausible, it requires further research and experiments. If it were to be corroborated, not only could the mirror mechanism be extended from observed actions to the space for action, but it would also be possible to confirm that the capacity to mirror the effective or potential actions of others depends primarily on the capacity to represent these actions motorically, as if they were being executed personally rather than just being seen to be executed by others.

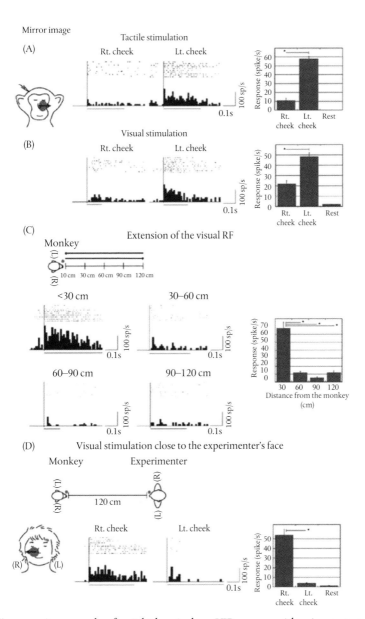

Fig. 2.14 An example of a right hemisphere VIP neuron with mirror properties for peripersonal space. (A, B) The neuron exhibited a tactile receptive field on the left cheek of the macaque and a visual receptive field located close to the same parts of the face. (C) Extension of the visual receptive field. The experimenter did not face the monkey. (D) Visual responses could be evoked by moving stimuli close to the experimenter's right cheek at 120 cm distance from the monkey (adapted from Ishida et al., 2010).

The Chapter in Brief

We have seen that mirror neurons can represent action *goals* such as grasping, kicking, climbing, etc. Observing this kind of action would evoke a transformation of the sensory representations concerning them into the motor representations of action goals similar to those that the observer would recruit if they themselves were to execute the observed actions (pp. 64–67).

The nature of this transformation explains why mirror responses are neither linked to individual visual aspects of the observed action nor to a single sensory modality. It also explains why they depend primarily on the capacity to represent action goals motorically. A number of studies show that the more this capacity develops, the greater the possibility of reflecting these goals when actions are observed rather than being executed (pp. 70–73).

There are two further points that should be kept well in mind. The *first* regards the discovery that mirror responses can be modulated by whether the observed actions are within or out of the observer's reach (pp. 76–80). The *second* is the discovery that there are mirror neurons that are able to encode both our own action space and that of others (pp. 80–83). In this case, the mirror mechanism would not entail the transformation of sensory representations concerning observed actions into motor representations of corresponding action goals; on the contrary, it would involve the transformation of representations of stimuli located in the peripersonal space of the individual being observed into motor representations of potential action goals—usually reach/grasp or avoid—similar to those which the observer would recruit if they themselves were to act on those stimuli, were they to appear in their peripersonal space. This is even more interesting because

84

certain neurons have been seen to combine mirror with canonical properties and that some of these respond not only while an action is being observed, but also when an object is presented that is out of the observer's reach, but only on the condition that it is located within reach, even potential reach, of another person.

Without a doubt, one of the most intriguing and promising areas for future research is the possibility that mirror neuron activity is not limited to the *actual* observation of an action; mirror neurons can also represent action goals that are merely *potential* for the observer. Indeed, Luca Bonini and colleagues at the University of Parma are working in that direction, having recorded the activity of single F5 neurons while a macaque was presented with a variant of the original task that requires executing a grasping action and observing the experimenter or another macaque doing the same (Bonini et al., 2014). This variant involved the addition of a cue specifying the action to be executed, followed by a Go or NoGo signal indicating whether the action was to be executed or inhibited, respectively. The result was quite unexpected. A portion of the recorded neurons fired even when the NoGo signal prevented the macaque from executing the cued action. Strikingly, mirror neurons were also found to fire not only when the cued action was actually observed, but also when the experimenter refrained from acting. It is interesting to note that the mirror responses were highly selective with respect to the action to be executed or inhibited and were mainly aligned with the NoGo signal. This suggests that the macaque recruited the same motor representations of one (or more) action goal(s) regardless of whether the cued actions were to be executed or not.

Another stimulating issue for future research concerns the possibility of integrating the study of the functional characteristics of the F5, PF/PFG, and AIP areas with the study of the functional properties of the various parietal, frontal, and prefrontal areas that recently have been shown to be endowed with the mirror property. It has been hypothesized that actions, whether executed personally or observed being executed by others, are represented by the activation of an extended network of areas (Gerbella et al., 2017). In fact, we have seen in Chapter 1 that mirror neurons have been recorded from the mesial frontal cortex, notably area F6 (pre-SMA), and the prefrontal areas (p. 10). We have also seen that area F6 hosts not only genuine mirror neurons, but also neurons that fire only when observing actions being executed by others (Yoshida et al., 2011; Livi et al., 2019). Given the reciprocal anatomical connections between these areas and those that constitute the core of the parieto-frontal network, and considering the respective functional properties which are similar in some cases and different in others (Lanzilotto et al., 2016; Simone et al., 2017), it would be most interesting to understand whether, and if so how, the various mirror responses might integrate with each other, thus contributing to motorically represent key aspects of the action being observed.

In this regard, it must be kept in mind that single cell recordings from area F6 have revealed mirror responses that appear to be linked to action targets. Indeed, neurons have been found that fired at the sight of objects that were targets of actions to be executed personally, neurons that fired at the sight of objects that were targets of actions to be executed by others, and lastly, neurons that fired in both conditions as long as the target objects were within the observer's reach (Livi et al., 2019). It would be of interest to assess whether, and if so how, F6 mirror responses and the corresponding sensorimotor transformations regarding action goals and targets are linked to the responses of F5 canonical, mirror, and canonical-mirror neurons. This could also shed new light on how the various parieto-frontal areas contribute to motorically representing peripersonal space, both our own and that of others, as action space.

CHAPTER 3

EMOTIONS

In Chapter 2 we explored the functional characteristics of mirror responses in the domain of action. We chose action as our starting point for historical and theoretic reasons: historical, as the mirror neurons were originally discovered in the premotor areas of the brain of the macaque; theoretic, because the study of mirror responses in the action domain has provided the basis on which to interpret their properties in other domains, including that of the emotions.[1] In this chapter we will focus on studies of mirror neuron responses while observing emotional expressions. We will show that these responses are specific to the observation of a certain kind of emotional reaction (such as disgust, fear, or laughter) and selectively involve a number of distinct brain centres (insula, amygdale, cingulate cortex).

---

[1] In the following pages we will use the terms emotion and emotional reaction in the pretheoretical sense in order to be as neutral as possible vis-à-vis the diverse conceptions of emotions to be found in the literature. We recommend Scarantino (2016) for further reading on this subject.

Mirroring Brains. Giacomo Rizzolatti and Corrado Sinigaglia, Oxford University Press. © Oxford University Press 2023. DOI: 10.1093/oso/9780198871705.003.0003

Emotion on your Face, and on Mine

The earliest studies suggesting the existence of mirror responses in the domain of emotions were carried out by Ulf Dimberg at the beginning of the 1980s. Basing his work on Charles Darwin's teachings, positing that basic emotions are expressed in specific facial patterns and body postures, Dimberg posed the question as to whether such patterns could be identified not only on the face of an individual experiencing a given emotion but also on the face of another individual observing that kind of emotion being expressed. In a seminal study in 1982, Dimberg recorded the EMG activity of the zygomatic major and upper corrugator in individuals observing static faces expressing happiness and anger. He found that observing happy faces results in an increase in this activity in the region of the zygomaticus major, while observing angry faces causes it to increase in the region of the upper corrugator. In Dimberg's own words, 'One interpretation of this is that subjects exposed to faces displaying a 'positive' or a 'negative' emotion, mirror EMG activity in facial muscle regions mediating 'positive' or 'negative' facial expressions, respectively' (Dimberg, 1982, pp. 645–646).

He replicated these results in later years, showing in particular that the EMG response is mainly automatic (Dimberg et al., 2002), can be connected to variations in heartbeat frequency or skin conductance (Dimberg, 1990), and occurs approximately 400 ms after the stimulus has appeared (Dimberg & Thunberg, 1998). In a study using a backward masking technique, Dimberg and colleagues presented their participants with an image of an angry, happy, or neutral (target stimulus) face for approximately 30 ms, followed by an image of an emotionally neutral face for approximately

5 sec (masked stimulus). By recording the EMG activity in the zygomaticus major and corrugator supercilii muscles, the authors found that even if their participants were not aware of the stimulus being presented (the target stimulus), they assumed a congruent facial expression: the corrugator supercilii was activated when observing an angry face, the zygomaticus major at the sight of a happy face.

The use of brain imaging techniques has opened the way for exploring cerebral activation while observing and imitating faces expressing positive and negative emotions. In an fMRI experiment in 2003, Marco Iacoboni and colleagues asked their participants to observe and imitate different emotional expressions (fear, disgust, anger, sadness, happiness, and surprise). Their results showed that the circuit involved in the motor control of facial expressions (posterior parietal cortex, inferior frontal gyrus) was also activated in the observation condition and that there was also activation in the anterior insula and the amygdala, two regions that are often activated when emotions are experienced rather than observed. They also found that the activation in these regions was greater when imitating facial expressions than when merely observing them. Similar results were also found in an fMRI experiment by a group of researchers led by Raymond Dolan and Hugo Critchley of University College London (Lee et al., 2006).

A Specific Mirror Mechanism for Emotions

How should these data be interpreted? Some researchers favour the hypothesis that premotor and motor areas endowed with the mirror property are primarily involved in a classic sensorimotor transformation by which visual representations of the facial expressions being observed are transformed into motor representations that come into play when we display these expressions ourselves.[2] Once the mirror mechanism is activated in the motor areas, the information relative to the facial expression being observed reaches centres such as the insula and the amygdala, triggering processes and representations with a specific emotional content. In other words, the transformations involved in mirror responses induced by observing emotional expressions in others, would be of the same kind as those active in mirror responses to actions of other people, the only difference being that in the first case, unlike the second, the motor representations would activate cortical or subcortical centres that give emotional colouring to a mirroring that *per se* is purely motoric.

However, without wishing to detract from the possible involvement of the parieto-frontal circuits, which as we have seen in Chapter 2 play a key role in the motor representation of actions such as grasping with the hand or the mouth that have no clear and characteristic emotional content, we feel there are solid grounds for supporting an alternative hypothesis according to which observing faces or body movements that express a given kind of emotion would directly activate brain centres involved in encoding that kind of emotion. This of course does not exclude that observing a face expressing an emotion or an emotionally charged body movement could also activate a mirror response of the motor areas. It must be kept in mind, however, that this is not the only mirror response possible, nor has it been found to have

---

[2] See, for example, Carr et al. (2003), Wood et al. (2016), de Waal and Preston (2017).

the properties necessary to capture the more specifically emotional aspects of the observed expression. In fact, capturing those aspects would primarily depend on the mirror responses of the brain centres that are involved in producing emotions.

So what is the rationale in support of this hypothesis? There are two points. First, the anatomy of the motor systems; studies on neurological patients have revealed the existence of two different motor systems, one being responsible for the execution and control of voluntary movements devoid of emotional content, the other for those of emotional reactions concerning the face and body posture (Holstege et al., 2004; Cattaneo & Pavesi, 2014). While the former is controlled by the primary motor cortex and the pyramidal tract, the latter is controlled by multiple centres including the insula, the amygdala, the cingulate gyrus, and their descending connections. In cases of paralysis, cortical lesions provoke a clear dissociation between these two systems. Patients with lesions in the cortical motor areas (or in their descending pathways) show a contralateral paralysis that frequently affects the mouth and prevents them from smiling voluntarily. However, if they are presented with a stimulus with comical content they smile in a normal manner (Ross, 1996; Waxman, 1996). On the contrary, there is evidence that patients with lesions primarily in the rostral area of the cingulate gyrus manage to smile voluntarily but are unable to smile or produce another emotional expression spontaneously (Gothard, 2014).[3]

---

[3] The fact that the two systems are separate for the most part does not mean they cannot interact. Take for example the possibility of voluntarily controlling, albeit within certain limits, facial or postural expressions provoked by disgust, fear, or mirth.

The second point concerns the pathways that underlie the processing of visual information regarding the features and expressions of the faces being observed. It has been known for some time that invariant features relevant for facial identity are processed by a ventral visual stream (called *the ventral stream for faces*) that includes visual areas V2–V4 and the inferior temporal region, while changeable features characteristic of various facial expressions are processed by a dorsal visual stream (*the dorsal stream for faces*) which is composed of the so-called middle-temporal area (MT) with its satellites and the areas of the superior temporal sulcus (STS) in the macaque and of analogous areas in humans (Furl et al., 2012; Bernstein & Yovel, 2015). The information regarding facial expressions undergoes further processing along another two streams: the motor information that characterizes all types of facial expressions is supposedly sent along the inferior parietal lobule (Rozzi et al., 2006) and the prefrontal ventral cortex (Deacon, 1992) to the premotor areas responsible for facial movements, while the information regarding the emotional characteristics of those expressions is delivered to various brain centres including the insula, the amygdala, and the anterior cingulate (Mufson & Mesulam, 1982; Morecraft et al., 2012).

In light of the above, the hypothesis of a purely motor mirror response, which would find a mere echo in a possible activation of brain centres like the insula and the amygdala, becomes highly unlikely. In addition, as we will see in the following chapters, there is convincing evidence that these brain centres are endowed with the mirror mechanism.

Unfortunately, apart from rare exceptions (Hutchison et al., 1999), there are no studies of recordings of single neurons in the two classic conditions of execution and observation from which to attribute the mirror property to the neurons of this or that area in the domain of the emotions, as there are in the domain of actions. Data regarding mirror responses that result from observing emotional facial expressions in others have been obtained mainly with brain imaging studies, in which it is fairly difficult to provoke emotional reactions so that they are both natural and controlled. In addition, as we will see in more detail later, while exposure to stimuli normally associated with a certain kind of emotional reaction results in a haemodynamic response, as is the response recorded with fMRI, this is not in itself sufficient in a cerebral area to attribute a precise emotion representation to that area (Mouraux et al., 2011; LeDoux & Brown, 2017). However, these limitations may be overcome by integrating brain imaging studies with others using different techniques (e.g. stereo-EEG) as well as by identifying the anatomical and functional characteristics by which a brain area can be considered to be involved in encoding a specific emotion. In the next section, we will show how at least three of these centres—specifically the anterior insula, the amygdala, and the anterior cingulate cortex—can be considered to be endowed with the mirror property.

Disgusted in the Insula

Mary Phillips and colleagues at King's College ran an fMRI study, published on *Nature* in October 1997, in which they showed their participants pictures of faces expressing two different levels of intensity of disgust. The participants were instructed simply to observe the pictures (Phillips et al., 1997; see also Phillips et al., 1998), which were then alternated with others showing faces with emotionally neutral expressions or expressions of fear with two levels of intensity. Analysis of the BOLD signal showed a clear activation of the anterior insular cortex that was not only selective for facial expressions of disgust but also incremented as the intensity of the disgust increased. Reiner Sprengelmeyer and colleagues at the University of Bochum obtained similar results when comparing cerebral responses to different kinds of emotional facial expressions. They found that when their participants observed facial expressions of disgust, there was a selective activation of the anterior insula (AI) and the right putamen (Sprengelmeyer et al., 1998).

Pierre Krolak-Salmon and colleagues at the University of Lyons implanted depth electrodes in drug-resistant epileptic patients during a presurgical evaluation process and recorded intracerebral event-related potentials (ERPs) to specific facial emotional expressions, including disgust (Krolak-Salmon et al., 2003). They found that while the patients were observing pictures of facial expressions of disgust there was a significant selective response of the ERPs recorded by the electrodes implanted in the ventral section of the AI, starting approximately 250–300 ms after the stimulus was presented.

Bruno Wicker and colleagues at the University of Marseilles and the University of Parma contributed significantly to attributing the mirror property to the AI with an experiment that, for the first time, showed evident overlapping in the activations of the AI induced by first-hand experience of disgust and by observing grimaces of disgust on the faces of other people (Wicker at al., 2003). This study was composed of two distinct sessions, one olfactory and one visual. In the first session, the participants were exposed to pleasant and unpleasant odours, while in the second they were asked to watch a number of videos in which an individual sniffed at glasses containing a liquid with an unpleasant smell, a pleasantly perfumed liquid, and an odourless liquid, making the appropriate facial expression. The participants did not know which kind of liquid was in the glass; their task was simply to observe the reaction of the person sniffing the liquid. The most interesting finding from this experiment was that not only did observation of facial expressions of disgust activate a portion of the AI, but also that this activation overlapped, albeit only partially, with the activation of AI induced by first-hand experience of unpleasant odours (Fig. 3.1).

This discovery was replicated and expanded on by Mbemba Jabbi and colleagues at the University of Groningen with an fMRI study during which they found a partial overlapping of AI activation in three different conditions: when the participants experienced disgust themselves, when they imagined experiencing it and lastly, when they saw disgust being expressed by others (Jabbi et al., 2007).

Given that the AI's response to the sight of a facial expression of disgust overlaps, albeit partially, with the response of the same portion of the insula induced by exposure to stimuli typically associated with experiencing disgust, there is good reason to claim that that particular portion of the insula is endowed with the mirror property. This claim seems to be corroborated by studies of electric macrostimulation of AI carried out on both monkeys and humans. A number of studies run in the 1950s have shown that when the AI is stimulated electrically, the animal produces a series of facial expressions and body movements that, unlike those induced by stimulation of the motor areas, are accompanied by a variety of visceral responses such as retching, variations in heartbeat,

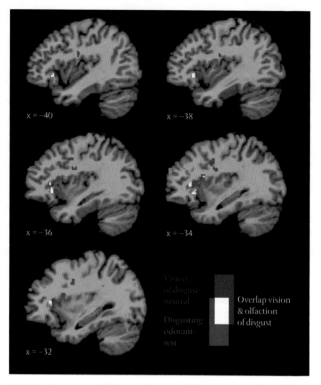

Fig. 3.1 Activations caused by unpleasant olfactory stimuli and the sight of faces expressing disgust. Brain activation at the sight of facial expressions of disgust is indicated in blue, while red indicates brain activation when experiencing unpleasant odours first-hand; white indicates the areas where the activations caused by both types of stimuli overlap. The results are superimposed on parasagittal slices of a standard MNI brain (adapted from Wicker et al., 2003).

dilation of the pupils, and so on (Kaada et al., 1949; Frontera, 1956; Showers & Lauer, 1961).

Much more recently, researchers of the Neuroscience Department of the University of Parma conducted two studies of intracortical microstimulation, showing that stimulation of the ventral sector of the AI in macaques results in motor and visceral reactions typical of disgust (Caruana et al., 2011; Jezzini et al., 2012) with classic grimaces such as raising the upper lip and wrinkling the nose, sometimes accompanied by bouts of retching. In certain cases the reactions were even more complex and articulated: for example, if the macaque was stimulated just as it was placing a grape or a peanut in its mouth, it would spit the food out instead of chewing it. If the stimulation was done while the monkey was taking food from the researcher, the animal would refuse it with an explicit arm gesture or, if the food was already in its hand, would throw it away. It is interesting that in both studies stimulation of the AI caused the heart rate to slow down significantly. While it is true that this effect can be associated with a number of states, it has been proved that disgust is the only negative emotion that causes it (Rozin et al., 2000).

Electric stimulation of AI evokes visceromotor reactions related to disgust in humans too; expressions of disgust and a strong sense of nausea have been recorded in drug-resistant epileptic patients when their insula was electrically stimulated by surgeons searching for a possible epileptic focus (Penfield & Faulk, 1955; Isnard et al., 2004). Similarly, Hélène Catenoix and colleagues (2008) reported the case of a patient in whom feelings of disgust were accompanied by bouts of vomiting during epileptic seizures when the AI was activated. Finally, we have already mentioned that Pierre Krolak-Salmon and colleagues found a significant ERP response recorded by electrodes implanted in the ventral portion of the AI while the patients were observing faces clearly expressing disgust. The authors also stimulated the same sites electrically, finding that almost all their patients complained of an unpleasant sensation that spread from the throat to the mouth and lips. Both ERPs and stimulation results suggest that the AI is endowed with the mirror property, playing a distinctive role in the detection of disgust in others and in feeling disgust oneself.

We saw in Chapter 1 that in both non-human primates and humans the AI contains a mosaic of bucco-facial behaviours ranging from ingestive actions (sited more dorsally) to disgust reactions (located more ventrally). Moreover, AI is known to be a visceromotor integration centre strongly connected with both olfactive and gustatory subcortical areas.[4] It also receives visual information from the anterior STS region, which in turn is connected to the MT area and its satellites. This network forms the so-called dorsal stream for faces, which is selectively involved in the representation of facial expressions, particularly those with emotional content (Furl et al., 2012; Bernstein & Yovel, 2015). With regard to the descending projections, AI projects to subcortical centres, such as the lateral hypothalamus, the ventral tegmental area, the ventral striate, and the ventro-lateral region of the periaqueductal gray (PAG), which modulate physiological responses while simultaneously controlling ingestive behaviour and visceromotor reactions (Fig. 3.2).[5]

Taken as a whole, the data cited above provide sound grounds for claiming that the ventral portion of AI is endowed with the mirror mechanism for disgust. In Chapter 2 we emphasized how mirror responses in the action domain involve a transformation of the sensory representations regarding the observed action into the motor representations of the possible goal(s) of that action (pp. 64–66). In Chapter 1 we saw that mirror responses vary

---

[4] See Mesulam and Mufson (1982a, 1982b), Mufson and Mesulam (1982), and Jezzini et al. (2015).

[5] See Öngür et al. (1998), An et al. (1998), Jezzini et al. (2015), Tremblay et al. (2015), and Venkatraman et al. (2017).

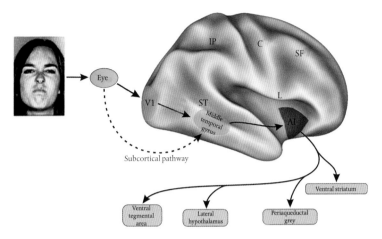

Fig. 3.2 The principal cortical and subcortical anatomical pathways by which the sight of a grimace of disgust reaches the subcortical and cortical centres, responsible for physiological, visceral, and motor responses typical of reactions of disgust when these are displayed in the first person.

Abbreviations: V1 = primary visual area, C = central sulcus, IP = intraparietal sulcus, L = lateral scissure, SF = superior frontal sulcus, ST = superior temporal sulcus, AI = anterior insula.

for the kinds of transformation achieved according to the functional characteristics of the various areas endowed with the mirror mechanism (p. 36). If we take the case of mirror responses from the AI, the data above suggest that these responses involve a transformation of the visual representations of the expressions of disgust seen on other people's faces into the motor and visceral processes and representations typically involved in our own experience of disgust. A goodly part of those visual representations come from the temporal lobe, so their transformation into visceromotor representations enables the information regarding the emotional body and facial expressions of others to access the same cortical and subcortical centres that are activated when the natural stimuli provoke the visceral and motor reactions typically related to reactions of disgust when we experience disgust ourselves.

Scared in the Amygdala

Another centre that appears to possess the mirror property is the amygdala. In the second half of the 1990s, Robert J. Dolan and colleagues studied the different neuronal responses evoked by the sight of facial expressions of fear or happiness. The data obtained from this study revealed a selective response in the left amygdala, which was not only greater for fearful facial expressions than for happy ones but actually increased with the intensity of the fear (Morris et al., 1996). Similarly, in an fMRI study Mary Phillips and colleagues discovered a selective activation of the left amygdala while their participants were viewing fearful expressions (Phillips et al., 1997). In a later study, they showed how the amygdala was selectively activated also by vocal expressions of fear (Phillips et al., 1998; see also Dolan et al., 2001). Along similar lines, while conducting an fMRI study at the Center for Biomedical Imaging of the Massachusetts General Hospital Nouchine Hadjikhani and Beatrice de Gelder found a haemodynamic response from the amygdala while their participants were viewing various bodily postures that clearly communicated a state of fear (Hadjikhani & de Gelder, 2003). Finally, Wataru Sato and colleagues at the University of Tokyo used fMRI to compare haemodynamic responses while their participants were viewing static and dynamic images representing fearful and happy faces (Sato et al., 2004). In both cases, viewing dynamic images entailed greater activation in cortical regions such as the inferior occipital gyrus, the medial-temporal gyrus, the fusiform gyrus, and the ventral premotor cortex, independently of whether the facial expressions were fearful or happy. On the other hand, only the sight of dynamic images representing facial expressions of fear induced more intense activation in the amygdala.

Taken together, these findings indicate that while the amygdala can respond to positive emotional expressions, it activates more intensely when viewing reactions and expressions of fear. Similar data were obtained from a series of intracranial recordings from patients with drug-resistant epilepsy (see for a review Murray et al., 2014). For example, Pierre Krolak-Salmon and colleagues discovered there was a much greater increase in the ERPs in the amygdala—occurring 200 ms after the stimulus was shown—when viewing faces expressing fear than when viewing happy or neutral faces (Krolak-Salmon et al., 2004). Wataru Sato and colleagues also found that viewing fearful faces evoked a greater response from the amygdala than viewing emotionally neutral faces (Sato et al., 2011). More recently Bryan Strange and colleagues at the University of Madrid (Méndez-Bértolo et al., 2016) recorded intracranial ERPs from electrodes implanted in the amygdala and the fusiform gyrus while their patients viewed images representing faces expressing fear, happiness, or no emotion whatsoever (neutral); these images were presented either in normal photographs or filtered so that only their low or high visual frequency components were visible. They found a selective amygdala activation for the fearful expressions; it was particularly interesting to see that the activation was extremely rapid (approximately 70 ms) when induced by fearful expressions with low frequency.

So far we have examined cases in which expressions of fear were observed on other people's faces. However, if we are to attribute the mirror property to the amygdala, especially in the case of reactions that are normally associated with fear, we have to ascertain if it has a role to play, and if so, what the role is, when we experience fear ourselves. Stefano Meletti and colleagues at the Universities of Bologna and Modena stimulated various areas of the temporal lobe, including the amygdala, the hippocampus, and the temporal cortex, in over seventy patients with drug-resistant epilepsy at Milan's Niguarda Hospital (Meletti et al., 2006). Stimulation varied by site, intensity, and frequency. The patients did not know where or when the stimulation would take place. Their reactions were classified according to evoked facial and vocal expressions as well as to bodily postures and verbal reports. The most interesting result was that the stimulation of the amygdala produced the greatest number of responses with emotional content, all of which consisted in expressions of fear as well as reports of experiencing anxiety and fear (see also Lanteaume et al., 2007 for similar data). More recently Cory Inman and colleagues stimulated the amygdala in a series of patients. They found a consistent pattern of physiological responses (modifications of skin conductance and heartbeat), which in a couple of cases were accompanied by feelings of anxiety and fear (Inman et al., 2018). It must be remembered that the induction of feelings of fear and anxiety were prevalent when stimulation was applied near the central nuclei of the amygdala.

As we pointed out in Chapter 1 (p. 27), the amygdala is a complex telencephalic structure. It receives information from the temporal and prefrontal regions responsible for processing complex social stimuli such as facial expressions and vocalizations (Amaral & Price, 1984; Gerbella et al., 2014). Its descending projections reach subcortical centres, such as the medial nuclei of the hypothalamus, the lateral region of the PAG, the locus coeruleus,

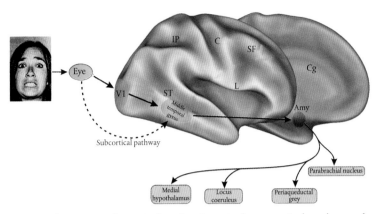

Fig. 3.3 The principal cortical and subcortical anatomical pathways by which the sight of a grimace of fear reaches the subcortical centres, responsible for physiological, visceral, and motor responses typical of reactions of fear when these are displayed in the first person.

Abbreviations: V1 = primary visual area, C = central sulcus, Cg = cingulate gyrus, IP = intraparietal sulcus, L = lateral sulcus, SF = superior frontal sulcus, ST = superior temporal sulcus, Amy = amygdala.

and the parabrachial nucleus that control the responses of the autonomous nervous system associated with defensive behaviour types of the fight-or-flight variety (Fig. 3.3).[6]

These findings suggest that the amygdala does possess the mirror property for those processes and representations that are typically involved in reactions to fear. Our hypothesis regarding what happens in the AI while observing expressions of disgust is equally applicable to the amygdala; here too the mirror responses entail a transformation of the visual and auditive representations of the fear we perceive in others, triggering the physiological, visceral, and motor responses typically associated with reactions of

---

[6] See Moga and Gray (1985), Price et al. (1987), An et al. (1998), and Motta et al. (2009).

fear and shaping the experience of fear when we experience it ourselves. Sensory representations come mainly from the temporal and prefrontal regions, and are transformed in the amygdala into visceromotor representations; as a consequence, information regarding the expressions of fear seen in other people is processed by the same subcortical and cortical circuits that are typically activated when reactions of fear are experienced personally.

Laughing in the Cingulate Gyrus

Recent research indicates that the anterior portion of the cingulate gyrus, and precisely the pregenual anterior cingulate, possesses the mirror property connected with laughter.

In spite of the fact that laughter plays a relevant social role with both emotional and communicative value, little is known about the cerebral areas and processes involved in laughing. The rare intracerebral studies conducted between the 1990s and the early 2000s showed that laughter can be evoked by stimulating cortical sites located in the rostral portion of the basal temporal lobe (Arroyo et al., 1993; Satow et al., 2003; Yamao et al., 2015) in the region that lies between the superior frontal gyrus and the supplementary motor area (Fried et al., 1998; Krolak-Salmon et al., 2006; Schmitt et al., 2006), in the opercular part of the inferior frontal gyrus (Férnandez-Baca Vaca et al., 2011), and in the anterior cingulate cortex (Sperli et al., 2006). However, all these studies involved a very limited number of participants (one, or a maximum of two) and the data available is not sufficient to establish the specific contribution of the areas involved, especially with regard to the more emotional aspects of laughter.

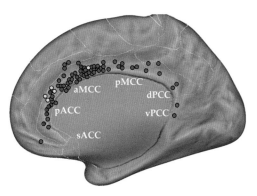

Fig. 3.4 Stimulated sites superimposed on a standard brain using CARET software. The yellow dots show the sites eliciting a burst of laughter, the red dots sites eliciting laughter without mirth. The black dots indicate sites eliciting other sensorimotor responses (adapted from Caruana et al., 2015).

Abbreviations: sACC = subgenual anterior cingulate cortex, pACC = pregenual anterior cingulate cortex, aMCC = anterior middle cingulate cortex, pMCC = posterior middle cingulate cortex, dPCC = dorsal posterior cingulate cortex, vPCC = ventral posterior cingulate cortex.

A significant step forward has been achieved with the recent study by Fausto Caruana and colleagues at the University of Parma (Caruana et al., 2015), in which over fifty drug-resistant epileptic patients from the Claudio Munari Center for Epilepsy Surgery of Milan's Niguarda Hospital participated. The most interesting finding of this study is related to the stimulation of the pregenual anterior cingulate cortex (pACC) (see Fig. 3.4).

When stimulated, approximately half of the patients suddenly burst out laughing, exhibiting an evident state of hilarity. The other half produced a timid smile, starting from the point on the face contralateral to where the stimulation was applied; they reported sensations located on the face but also on the neck and in other parts of the body (Fig. 3.5).

Apart from the usual differences in the patients' responses, due to their personality traits as well as probably to the different

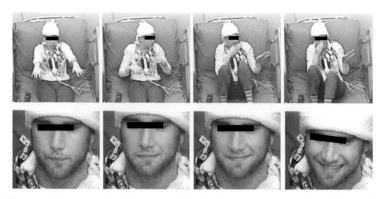

Fig. 3.5 Upper panel: When stimulated, the patient immediately stopped reading and burst out laughing. She said that she had felt an irresistible impulse to laugh that she could not explain. Lower panel: low intensity stimulation elicited a smile from the patient, starting from the contralateral zygomaticus and the orbicularis oculi muscles, then spreading to the entire face, and eventually producing a wide smile (adapted from Caruana et al., 2015).

stimulation sites (those which induced laughter and hilarity tended to be located in the more caudal and dorsal portion of the pACC, see Fig. 3.4), the results obtained by Fausto Caruana and colleagues indicate that processes and representations take place in the pACC that can trigger motor and visceromotor reactions with a specific emotional valence, such as a mirthful laugh.

A group of researchers led by Kendall H. Lee of the Mayo Clinic in Rochester (USA) obtained similar results from a study combining deep brain stimulation (DBS) and fMRI (Gibson et al., 2016). DBS of the ventral portion of the internal capsule and the ventral striate is an FDA-approved therapy for the treatment of compulsive-obsessive disorders in drug-resistant patients (Greenberg et al., 2010); clinical testing has shown that it can modify states of mind, making patients more cheerful and inducing them to smile, even to burst out laughing. By stimulating a number of patients and analysing the consequent change in the BOLD signal, Kendall Lee and colleagues found a significant modulation of the pACC, and more importantly, they saw that this modulation only occurred when the stimulation induced hilarity and laughter.

Masahiro Matsunaga and colleagues at the Aichi Medical University School of Medicine in Japan worked along the same lines with a study that showed how the rostral cingulate cortex is structurally and functionally associated with personality traits and states of mind, both characterized by a positive emotional valence (Matsunaga et al., 2016). Using a technique known as *voxel-based morphometry* that applies parametric statistical mapping to examine focal differences in the brain's anatomy by individual voxel, the authors not only found that the activation of the rostral cingulate cortex changed with variations in the positive state of mind but also that the activation correlated with the density of the grey matter in that location.

Taken together, these studies show that not only does the pACC control the purely motor aspects of laughter as has been suggested in the past (see, for example, Arroyo et al., 1993; Satow et al., 2003; Sperli et al., 2006), it also contributes to processing the visceral and emotional aspects.[7] So far we have focused on the pACC's contribution to our own laughter and mirth, and have not yet mentioned

---

[7] These results contribute to a preliminary draft of a first brain map of laughter that takes includes its various forms and goes beyond dichotomies such as those of 'motor' laughter and 'emotional' laughter. The reader will remember that, when stimulated, the basal temporal lobe evokes laughter which may be accompanied by a feeling of hilarity. We know that this region sends input to the rostral portion of ACC and, even more importantly, that it is involved in processing semantic information and in high-order memory processes. This leads to the hypothesis that it plays a role in codifying the incongruencies typical of humoristic jokes (Vrticka et al., 2013). Other sites, such as the supplementary motor area and the frontal operculum, are also connected to the pACC (Luppino et al., 1993; Gerbella

the most important aspect for the purposes of this book: the pACC has been seen to be endowed with the mirror property, responding also when other people laugh and manifest hilarity.

Diana P. Szameitat and colleagues at the University of Tübingen ran an fMRI study in which the participants were asked to listen to laughter that had a clear emotional valence (joyous or humorous) or which was induced by tickling (Szameitat et al., 2010). Their results showed an activation of the anterior cingulate gyrus selective for laughter with an emotional valence, whereas laughter as a consequence of tickling elicited a stronger response in the median region of the temporal superior gyrus, which is typically involved in the coding of complex acoustic stimuli without any specific emotional content. These results are supported by a meta-analysis of over one hundred fMRI studies concerning the visual perception of emotional faces, which revealed that when observing faces expressing happiness compared to faces with neutral expressions, the pACC activated selectively (Fusar-Poli et al., 2009). This would suggest that under normal circumstances and independently of the sensory modality involved, the pACC conveys information regarding observed laughter and related emotional behaviours.

The most convincing evidence to support the hypothesis that the pACC might have the mirror property is to be found in a recent study conducted by Fausto Caruana and colleagues, in which they combined electrical stimulation and intracranial electroencephalogram recordings in a patient with drug-resistant focal epilepsy. The authors showed the patient a number of video-clips illustrating an actor laughing, crying, and expressing no emotion

et al., 2016), though it is plausible that they play a role prevalently in the circuit for spontaneous laughter (Caruana et al., 2015).

whatsoever. As in the previous studies, stimulating the pACC elicited a smile. The sites that evoked laughter showed an increase of gamma band activity (50–100 Hz) only while the patient was watching the video-clip showing the actor laughing. No significant effect was reported while the patient was watching the video-clips of the actor crying, or not expressing any emotion (Fig. 3.6).

For a better understanding of these data, it must be remembered that in the macaque, the homologous portion of the anterior cingulate gyrus is connected with the caudal raphe nucleus, a brainstem structure that, when damaged, may produce the phenomenon of uncontrolled laughter in humans known as *fou rire prodromique* (Hornung, 2003). In addition, projections descending from the pACC reach the portion of the putamen that controls

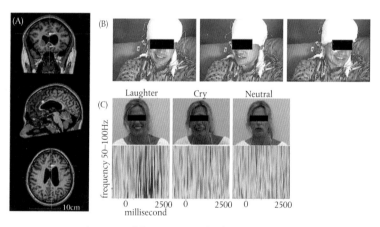

Fig. 3.6 (A) Localization of the contacts which produced a smile when stimulated electrically. The yellow dots indicate the internal contact employed for stimulation and intracranial recording. (B) Facial expression elicited by electric stimulation of the pACC (50 Hz, 5 s, 2 mA). (C) Time-frequency maps showing gamma band modulation while observing a person laughing, crying, and with a neutral expression (adapted from Caruana et al., 2017).

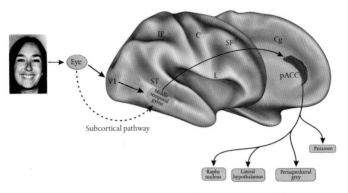

Fig. 3.7 The principal anatomical cortical and subcortical pathways along which observation of a laughing face reaches the cortical and subcortical centres responsible for physiological, visceral, and motor responses that are typically recruited when laughing.

Abbreviations: V1 = primary visual area, C = central sulcus, Cg = cingulate sulcus, IP = intraparietal sulcus, L = lateral scissure, SF = superior frontal sulcus, LF = lateral frontal sulcus, ST = superior temporal sulcus, pACC = pregenual anterior cingulate cortex, Cg = cingulate sulcus.

hand and mouth movements, the ventral striate which is typically involved in behaviour producing pleasure and reward, the vocalization centres localized in the dorsolateral portion of the PAG, and the nuclei of the facial nerves.[8] These latter projections channel information to the dorsal and intermediate subdivisions of the facial nerve nucleus, thus controlling the upper facial muscles that are involved in the act of laughing, particularly when it has a specific emotional valence as in the case of mirthful laughter (Fig. 3.7).

Finally, like the insula and the amygdala, the pACC is connected to the anterior region of the STS. From this area and from the

---

[8] See Müller-Preuss and Jürgens (1976), Porrino and Goldman-Rakic (1982), Devinsky et al. (1995), An et al. (1998), and Morecraft et al. (2001).

medial-temporal area with which it is connected, the pACC receives visual information regarding emotional facial expressions (Furl et al., 2012; Bernstein & Yovel, 2015).

This indicates that when we observe smiling faces, the mirror responses in the pACC transform the visual representations of those smiles into visceral and motor processes and representations similar to those we would recruit if we were laughing ourselves. Therefore our earlier comments regarding visceromotor transformations evoked by the mirror responses of the AI and the amygdala are also applicable to the pACC: the sensory representations arrive principally from the temporal regions and their transformation in the pACC into visceromotor representations allows the information regarding other people's expressions of laughter and mirth to be processed by the same cortical and subcortical circuits that are usually activated by our own smiling or bouts of laughter, accompanied by a more or less pronounced feeling of mirth.

Ready to act in the Cingulate Gyrus

We have already mentioned how the first mirror neurons discovered in humans were recorded in the anterior portion of the middle cingulate cortex (aMCC), situated rostrally on the plane that passes through the anterior commissure. At the end of the 1990s, William Duncan Hutchison and colleagues at the University of Toronto studied the activity of single neurons in patients undergoing bilateral cingulotomy for therapeutic purposes. Their objective was to identify the portions of the cingulate cortex responding to painful stimuli. For this purpose, the surgeons applied very cold or very hot stimuli or used nociceptive mechanical stimuli such as pricking with a needle or pinching skin between fingers. Approximately one-sixth of the neurons recorded in the aMCC (11/68) responded to these latter stimuli, and most of them responded selectively either to the thermal or the mechanical nociceptive, while others responded to both. None of the recorded neurons responded to neutral stimuli, such as a simple touch (Hutchison et al., 1999).

The most important finding from this study was that neurons that responded selectively when a patient was pricked with a needle also activated when the patient saw the experimenter being similarly pricked (Fig. 3.8).

A few years later, Tania Singer and colleagues at University College London conducted an fMRI study comparing the haemodynamic responses of sixteen couples while being subjected to a painful stimulus and while observing the same stimulus being applied to others (Singer et al., 2004). More precisely, the authors recorded the cerebral activity of sixteen women when a painful stimulus was applied to the back of their hands and when a similar stimulus was applied to their partners. Their results showed that in the aMCC there was a clear overlapping of the activations induced by the painful stimulus applied to the participants and of the activations induced by observing the same stimulus applied to their partners.

How should these data be interpreted? Taken as a whole, they suggest that the aMCC, or at least a part of it, possesses the mirror property. However, it is not yet clear what the mirror responses recorded in this area actually 'mirror'. The hypothesis that immediately comes to mind is that they are mirroring the reaction to pain

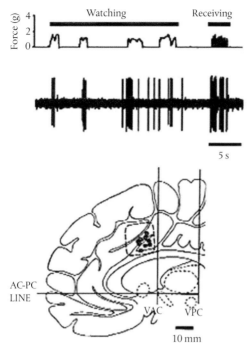

Fig. 3.8 Above: an aMCC neuron that responded both to the sight of nociceptive stimuli applied to the experimenter (left) and to the patient (right). Below: a diagram of a sagittal view illustrating the location of the recorded neurons that responded to nociceptive stimuli.

Abbreviations: VAC = vertical line through the anterior commissure, VPC = vertical line through the posterior commissure (adapted from Hutchison et al., 1999).

being suffered by another person. If this is in fact the case, it would mean that watching another person being subjected to a painful stimulus determines, in the observer's brain, the transformation of the sensory representations relative to the stimulation of others into the representations and the processes that typically trigger the reactions to our own feelings of pain. This hypothesis seems to be supported by brain imaging studies in which thermal and mechanical nociceptive stimuli were used to activate the aMCC.[9] Indeed, these studies led some researchers to believe that the aMCC is a key region in the so-called 'neuromatrix of pain' (Melzack, 2001, 2005) and is selectively involved in the representation of the more affective aspects of experiencing pain (Rainville et al., 1997). Not surprisingly, in their fMRI study mentioned above Tania Singer and colleagues noted that observing other people's pain did not recruit the entire 'neuromatrix of pain' as the somatosensory cortices and the posterior portion of the insula only responded to the painful stimulus when experienced personally. The fact that the aMCC also responded when this stimulus was applied to others had led them to surmise that observing other people's pain activated the affective, not the sensory, component of the neuromatrix.

It is certainly not our intention to enter into a discussion of the *vexata quaestio* regarding the putative existence of a cerebral matrix of pain.[10] We are only interested here in understanding whether the aMCC mirror responses are selective for other people's pain and if so, whether the transformations that they trigger regard processes and representations typically involved in reactions to and experience of pain. Indeed, there is more than one reason for believing that this is not the case.

---

[9] See Peyron et al. (2000) and Vogt (2005) for a meta-analysis of the fMRI and PET data.

[10] There is a vast literature dealing with the possible existence of a network of cortices (such as the primary and secondary somatosensory cortices, and the cortices of the cingulate and the insula) specifically involved in the perception of pain, which has been named the 'neuromatrix of pain'. For further reading regarding the brain imaging data supporting this hypothesis, see Ingvar (1999), Peyron et al. (2000), Porro (2003), Rainville (2002), Tracey and Mantyh (2007), Vogt and Sikes (2009), and Wager et al. (2013), among others. A rich and articulate critique of the 'neuromatrix of pain' hypothesis and an alternative interpretation of the data has been formulated by Legrain et al. (2011) and Iannetti et al. (2013), among others.

First of all, it must be remembered that William Hutchinson and colleagues not only recorded the activity of the aMCC neurons while painful stimuli were being applied to their participants; they also electrically stimulated the sites from which the neurons were recorded. To their surprise, however, none of the sites they stimulated elicited unpleasant sensations or pain, even when high voltage stimuli were used. The absence of pain when stimulating the sites of the neurons activated by specific nociceptive stimuli led these authors to hypothesize that, among other things, these neurons could have an important role to play in mediating behaviours that may be associated with the experience of pain, but do not necessarily coincide with it. Regarding this aspect, the fact that a portion of the recorded neurons responded selectively when anticipating a potentially painful stimulus or just watching it, is in itself significant.[11]

It becomes even more significant when compared with the results Akichika Mikami and colleagues at the University of Kyoto obtained from their experiments with macaques (Koyama et al., 1998). They recorded the activity of single aMCC neurons while the animal was engaged with a pain-avoidance task consisting in releasing a lever on the appearance of a signal that preceded the possibility of a reward or a slightly painful shock. The results showed that a portion of the recorded neurons responded selectively when the signal threatening the electric shock appeared; after just a few trials the animal was able to avoid the electric shock, releasing the lever in time. Only approximately fifty per cent of these neurons also responded when the nociceptive stimulus was actually

[11] The representation and processing of nociceptive stimuli do not necessarily entail that pain will be felt (Baumgärtner et al., 2006; Lee et al., 2009), and indeed there are data showing that pain can be experienced in the absence of nociceptive stimuli (Nikolajsen & Jensen, 2006).

applied. The authors concluded that the macaque's aMCC possesses neurons that codify the anticipation of a potential threat, which does not itself entail any painful sensation and allows the animal to trigger avoidance or flight behaviour according to the context (see also Koyama et al., 2001).

Taken together, these data would suggest that rather than being related to pain itself, the aMCC responds to the possibility of a threat that is more or less likely to materialize, triggering the appropriate motor behaviour. At this point it is interesting to remember that as early as 1973 Jean Talairach and colleagues at the Sainte-Anne Hospital Center of Paris had observed that electric stimulation of aMCC sites located rostrally on the plane that passes through the anterior commissure evoked a series of highly integrated motor behaviours. These behaviours could involve either the whole body or, as was more often the case, just the upper limbs. When involving the latter, they resulted in grasping actions directed away from the body or body-directed reaching and rubbing actions; it is relevant that none of these responses had affective content or expressed any kind of emotion (Talairach et al., 1973).

Similar results were obtained recently by Giacomo Rizzolatti and colleagues in a study conducted in collaboration with the Claudio Munari Center for Epilepsy Surgery of Milan's Niguarda Hospital. The study involved 300 patients and almost 1800 stimulated sites, aiming at a detailed mapping of the cingulate cortex (Caruana et al., 2018). The most interesting result for the purposes of this book is that the majority of the stimulations applied to the aMCC triggered an aggregate of complex motor behaviours most of which were executed fluidly and naturally, all having the characteristics of goal-directed behaviour (Fig. 3.9). For example, when stimulated, patients made postural adjustments that clearly

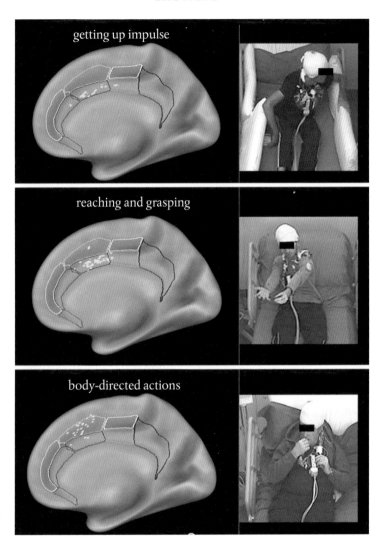

Fig. 3.9 Three main goal-directed behavioural responses elicited by stimulation of the aMCC. The left panel depicts the anatomical location of the stimulated sites relative to each behaviour (adapted from Caruana et al., 2018).

indicated an impellent need to get up from the bed and leave the room; a number of patients even reported having felt this need at the very moment when the stimulation was applied. In other cases, stimulation of the aMCC elicited reaching and grasping actions, even when there were no objects to be reached for or grasped, while in others it elicited exploratory movements of the eyes and of the head. Part of the motor behaviour induced by the stimulation consisted in body-directed actions, particularly to the face; the patients rubbed their eyes, tried to remove something from their mouths or simply tried to protect their face with their hands.

It is important to note that, as in Jean Talairach's study, no actual feelings of pain were caused by stimulation of the aMCC. This finding is corroborated by an fMRI study conducted by Gian Domenico Iannetti and colleagues at University College London (Mouraux et al., 2011) in which they compared the activations elicited by a random sequence of brief nociceptive somatosensory, non-nociceptive somatosensory, auditory, and visual stimuli. The results showed a clear overlapping in the aMCC of the activations elicited by the four different kinds of stimuli; in addition, the activations were stronger when the participants considered the stimuli to be salient. The authors concluded that activation of the aMCC principally reflects processes and representations that are essential to orient attention to generally salient stimuli, to assess the potential threat or undesirability they pose and when necessary, to trigger the appropriate behavioural response.[12]

[12] This conclusion is compatible with the results obtained from several fMRI studies, in which the aMCC has been seen to be activated in a series of purely cognitive tasks such as the Stroop and Eriksen-Flanker tasks and their variants, as well as the classic Go/NoGo tasks. These tasks also test the capacity to respond adequately to salient conflicting stimuli—for example, a word indicating a colour (the word 'red', for example) written with either a congruent (red) or an

It is worth noting that the aMCC projects both to the reticulo-spinal tract and to the spinal roof tract. While the reticulospinal tract is responsible for controlling proximal movements (postural adjustments, locomotion, etc.; Kuypers, 1981) and distal movements (reaching, grasping, etc.; Honeycutt et al., 2013), the spinal roof tract is responsible for head and eye movements and their coordination with the distal movements of the upper limbs (Leichnetz et al., 1981; May, 2006). The descending projections of the aMCC reach the portions of the putamen involved in controlling limb movements; they also reach the longitudinal column of the PAG, which is mainly involved in the motor production of the most natural defence mechanisms when threatened (An et al., 1998). Last but not least, the aMCC is not only one of the main cortical targets of the spinothalamic pathway responsible for the transmission of nociceptive information, it also functions as a 'bridge' to the motor system (Dum et al., 2009) as it is connected to the spinal cord and red nucleus (Luppino et al., 1994) as well as to the dorsal premotor (Dum & Strick, 2005) and mesial supplementary motor cortices (Luppino et al., 1993) (Fig. 3.10).

If we combine the anatomical and functional properties of the aMCC described earlier, it is clear that this portion of the cingulate cortex plays a distinctive role in transforming a great variety of stimuli into a collection of highly integrated and complex motor responses implementing defensive or aversive behaviours to an apparent threat, or simply to something that is perceived as unpleasant or undesirable.

incongruent (red) colour; an arrow or a letter flanked by other arrows or letters potentially causing interference; a Go/NoGo signal. A meta-analysis of aMCC activations in cognitive control tasks can be found in Nee et al. (2007) and Shackman et al. (2011).

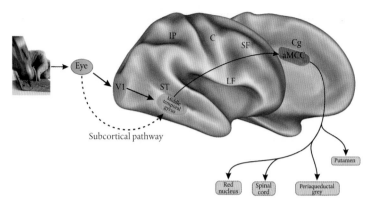

Fig. 3.10 The observation of a stimulus potentially or really threatening for another person passes along these main cortical and subcortical pathways to reach the central cortices responsible for inducing a state of alert and triggering a correspondent motor behaviour when this kind of threat is experienced personally.

Abbreviations: V1 = primary visual area, ST = superior temporal sulcus, IP = intraparietal sulcus, C = central sulcus, SF = superior frontal sulcus, L= lateral scissure, aMCC anterior middle cingulate cortex, Cg = cingulate sulcus.

This allows us to make a provisional characterization of the kind of transformation involved in the aMCC mirror responses. The sensory representations evoked by observing another person being subjected to a possibly painful stimulus or exposed to something that can be perceived as potentially threatening, would be transformed into the motor representations that normally trigger a state of alertness and prepare appropriate motor behaviour when these stimuli are processed and possibly perceived at first hand. This sensorimotor transformation enables information regarding the kind of stimulus being experienced by another person, whether painful or not, to be processed by the same cortical and subcortical circuits that play a key role in directing attention, in recognizing possible threats or harmful situations and triggering the cascade of appropriate motor behaviours when the observer themselves experience that kind of stimulus.

The Chapter in Brief

In this chapter we have seen that mirror responses are not the pre-rogative of the cerebral areas involved in the motor representation of action. Observing a grimace of disgust can trigger a mirror response in the anterior portion of the insula that is known to act as a visceromotor integration centre, involved in representing the visceral and motor reactions that contribute to forming the personal experience of disgust. The same holds true for observing facial expressions or bodily movements registering fear that can find a mirror response in the amygdala, a complex telencephalic structure involved in the representation of physiological and motor reactions normally associated with fear when it is experienced personally. Finally, seeing a cheerful smile can evoke the mirror response of the pACC, a portion of the cingulate cortex; activation of this area is linked to a complex pattern of visceral and motor responses typical of laughter, especially of mirthful laughter.

In all three cases, the mirror responses entail a sensorimotor and visceromotor transformation that changes according to the areas involved. Where AI mirror responses are concerned, the sensory representations of a grimace of disgust are transformed into the visceromotor representations which, if evoked by personal exposure to natural stimuli such as unpleasant smells or flavours, trigger reactions typical of disgust. Similarly, if we consider the amygdala, the sensory representations of expressions of fear observed in other people are transformed into the visceromotor representations which normally result from exposure to threatening stimuli experienced personally, triggering typical reactions of fear. Lastly, the same holds true for sensory representations of other people's laughter that are transformed into the visceromotor representations that contribute to making us laugh ourselves, and may be accompanied by a sense of mirth that may vary in intensity. The mirror responses of the aMCC are different, but nonetheless interesting. Our hypothesis is that this response represents a motor state of alert or readiness induced by an impending threat, rather than by an actually painful experience.

As we have seen, a great deal of data has been collected and numerous studies have been conducted on the mirroring of emotions over the last fifteen years. There is no doubt, however, that much still remains to be done in order to fully understand how the mirror mechanism works in the emotion domain.

One of the most interesting issues, and certainly most promising for future research, is whether mirror responses might be related to emotional behaviours that are more complex than a simple grimace of disgust or of fear. A few years ago, Nicola Canessa and colleagues at Milan's San Raffaele University and the University of Parma took a step in that direction. They recorded changes in the haematic flow of subjects professing a feeling of regret themselves and when they observed others experiencing a similar feeling (Canessa et al., 2009). Regret is considered to be a complex, cognitively based negative emotional reaction as it presupposes the capacity to take responsibility for choices made, and to make counterfactual reflections on the alternatives and the possible benefits that could accrue from selecting one particular choice rather than another. In Nicola Canessa's study, the participants were asked to bet on one of two options, one involving a real win and the other an equally real loss, and watch others doing the same; once the results of the bets were revealed, they were asked to indicate whether they were satisfied with their bet, and also whether in their opinion the other players were satisfied with the outcome of their choices. The study included a control condition, in which the bets were placed randomly by a computer; in this case, as the participants felt no responsibility for the bet, the resulting emotion was not regret, but simply disappointment. Analysis of the BOLD signal revealed activation of the ventromedial prefrontal cortex, the dorsal portion of the central cingulate gyrus and the hippocampus, both when the participants regretted their own choice and when they judged that others were experiencing the same feeling.

If these findings suggest the existence of mirror responses selective for a complex emotion such as regret, should also we expect something similar from observing expressions of social emotions such as jealousy or shame? Are there grounds to suppose that there will be selective mirror responses for these expressions too? Assuming that this is the case, which transformation would be involved? These are just a few of the questions that need to be answered. It is to be hoped that future research will soon provide a more detailed picture of the brain areas responding to emotional expressions, as well as of the processes and representations involved in their mirror responses.

CHAPTER 4

VITALITY FORMS

U p to now, we have limited our considerations to actions and emotional expressions, deliberately avoiding touching on the affective components that appear to be inextricably part of them. Whatever the goals of your actions, they may be *energetic, firm, decisive*, sometimes even *rigid* or *contracted*, but they can also be *hesitant, relaxed*, or *effortless*. You can pick up that glass *rudely* or *carelessly, energetically*, or *delicately*, just as you can shake a friend's hand *warmly*, or that of a person you are meeting for the first time *warily, forcefully, hesitantly, quickly*, or *kindly*. The same can be said of your emotional reactions: you can experience an *irrepressible* or *slight* sense of disgust, a spurt of *explosive* or *repressed* anger, your face can be contorted in a *terrible* scowl or a *fleeting* grimace.

Daniel Stern pointed out that people mainly use adjectives or adverbs when expressing themselves in these terms. But what do these adjectives and adverbs refer to? According to Stern,

> the items [. . .] are not emotions. They are not sensations in the strict sense, as they have no modality. They are not cognitions in any usual sense. They are not acts, as they have no goal state and no specific means. [. . .] They are more *form* than *content*. They concern the 'How', the manner, and the style, not the 'What' or the 'Why'. (Stern, 2010, pp. 9–11; our italics)

Mirroring Brains. Giacomo Rizzolatti and Corrado Sinigaglia, Oxford University Press. © Oxford University Press 2023. DOI: 10.1093/oso/9780198871705.003.0004

Adjectives and adverbs refer to the *dynamic forms* that characterize actions and emotional expressions (such as a *rude* rather than *limp* handshake, or *cold* anger rather than *explosive* wrath) regardless of their content (*grasping* rather than *kicking*, a grimace of *disgust* rather than *fear*). Stern himself, in the course of his long career, assigned various labels to these dynamic forms such as 'profiles', 'affects', or 'vitality forms' (Stern, 1985, 2004, 2010).

Stern's concept of vitality forms has twofold relevance for the purposes of this book. First, it posits that no action or emotional expression exists without being qualified by a vitality form and that the differences between the various vitality forms cannot be interpreted in terms of difference of content. In particular, as Stern has often emphasized, the differences between vitality forms are not the same as differences between emotions, since the same kind of emotion can be expressed in different forms and conversely, the same form can identify different kinds of emotion (Stern, 2010, pp. 24–25, 38–39). This means, among other things, that to fully understand how actions and emotions are represented at the cerebral level it is necessary to factor in different processes and representations from those that have been considered up to now. Furthermore, they should be computed by brain areas other than those involved in controlling actions and emotions, albeit still connected with them. These processes and representations execute their own specific function, which is to shape the activity of the areas involved in controlling actions and emotions so as to mould this or that *content* with this or that *form*.

Secondly, in Stern's view, the capacity of representing one's own vitality forms and those of others plays a key role in the appearance and development of various forms of intersubjectivity. This role is more important and fundamental than that which is usually ascribed to representing our own actions or emotional expressions and those of others. According to Stern, in fact, 'sharing vitality forms' represents the 'oldest, most direct and immediate' modality of 'affective tuning' with others, and is so 'deeply rooted' and 'natural' as to pervade every social interaction (Stern, 2010, pp. 31 and following).[1]

Surprisingly, in spite of their importance and pervasiveness, vitality forms have been almost totally ignored by cognitive neuroscience.[2] That is not to say that nothing has been done to explore the neural correlates of the important components of affectivity over the last two decades,[3] but until recently there was very little research done on brain areas underlying the processing of vitality forms.

---

[1] This view is largely shared by many authors including Colwyn Trevarthen (1998), Philippe Rochat (1999, 2009), and Stein Bråten (1998).

[2] Stern himself attributed this state of affairs to the very pervasiveness of the forms of vitality, however paradoxical that may seem: 'How is it that dynamic forms of vitality are relatively little considered and understood? We know them so well, perhaps too well. Forms of vitality are hard to grasp because we experience them in almost all waking activities. They are obscured by the felt quality of emotions as it accompanies them. [. . .] It is strange that even when it comes to motor acts, dynamic experiences are most often taken for granted as a part of means-end operations to accomplish a goal, and thus receive little additional attention' (Stern, 2010, p. 10).

[3] There is no doubt that today affective neuroscience is one of the richest and most interesting fields of research and that Jaak Panksepp has contributed to this success. We recommend Panksepp (1998) and Panksepp and Biven (2012) for further reading and Armony and Vuillemier (2013) for an introduction to affective neuroscience.

Hand action vitality forms

Thanks to the collaboration with Stern, over the last five years or so our group has started an in-depth study of the cerebral areas specifically involved in the representation of our own vitality forms and those of others, with a particular focus on action vitality forms.

In these studies, one of the problems we have encountered is how to disentangle the form from the content. Take the example of grasping a glass rudely or gently; how can the rudeness or gentleness in our grasping be disentangled from the actual grasping? One way of doing this is to vary the kind of vitality form (i.e. *rude* versus *gentle*) while keeping the action goal (*grasping*) as a constant; and vice versa, in varying the kind of action goal (*grasping* versus *giving*), while maintaining the vitality form (*gentle*) as a constant.

By adopting this strategy, Giuseppe Di Cesare and colleagues at the University of Parma, working together with Daniel Stern, conducted an fMRI study in which participants were presented with video clips showing four transitive actions (e.g. grasping a cup, giving a packet of crackers: Fig. 4.1A) and four intransitive actions (e.g. shaking hands, stopping gestures: Fig. 4.1B). All the actions were performed with two different vitality forms (gentle and rude). The participants were shown the stimuli in pairs of consecutive video clips, in which the goal of the observed action and its vitality form could either remain the same or change between the video pairs. There were two tasks, *What* and *How*; in the *What* task, the participants were asked to concentrate on the aim of the actions observed in the two consecutive video clips and decide

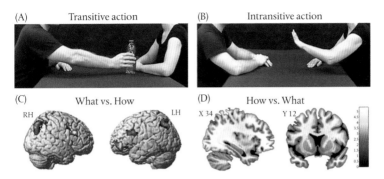

Fig. 4.1 Example of video clips shown to participants illustrating a transitive action (passing a bottle) (A) or an intransitive action (stop gesture) (B). Brain activations resulting from the contrast between the *What* task and the *How* task (C) and the *How* task and the *What* task (D) (adapted from Di Cesare et al., 2014).

whether the two action goals were the same or different, regardless of their vitality form, while in the *How* task, they were required to focus their attention on the action vitality form and to decide whether it was the same or different in the two video clips, regardless of which action goal was achieved.

In both tasks, the results showed activations, stronger for the *What* task, in the parieto-frontal network known to be involved in the observation and execution of actions relative to the *How* task, in the ventral premotor cortex, in the posterior parietal lobe bilaterally, and in the inferior frontal gyrus of the left hemisphere (Fig. 4.1C). Most importantly, contrasting the *How* task versus the *What* task revealed a specific activation in the right dorso-central insula (DCI) (Fig. 4.1D). We had expected to find activation of the parieto-frontal circuit during action observation (see Chapter 2, pp. 53–60), but the activation of the DCI during action vitality form observation was the first demonstration that this sector of the insula plays a specific role in processing action vitality forms (Di Cesare et al., 2014).

In a subsequent fMRI study, Di Cesare and colleagues took a step further in investigating the neuronal underpinning of vitality forms by asking participants not only to observe, but also to execute and imagine actions such as picking up and passing a bottle to another person, using two different vitality forms, gentle and rude (Di Cesare et al., 2015). As a control condition, participants had to observe a hand placing a small ball inside a box, to imagine themselves executing the same action, and then execute that action themselves without any particular vitality form (Fig. 4.2).

As was to be expected, activation of the parieto-frontal areas was found in all three conditions. As explained in Chapter 2, these areas are involved in the representation of the action goal, whether imagined, observed, or actually executed. An important finding emerged from the comparison between the three conditions in which the vitality forms of the observed, imagined, and executed actions and the control condition in which there was no manipulation of the vitality form varied; as can be seen in Fig. 4.3, this comparison revealed significant activation of the DCI during the observation, imagination, and executions of actions performed with different vitality forms.

The conjunction analysis on the activations in all three conditions showed bilateral activation in the premotor and parietal cortices, and a strong activation of the left somatosensory cortex, motor cortex, and the dorsal part of the cerebellum for both vitality forms (gentle and rude). Importantly the analysis also revealed a strong activation of the DCI, thus suggesting that this portion of the insula possesses the mirror property (Fig. 4.4).

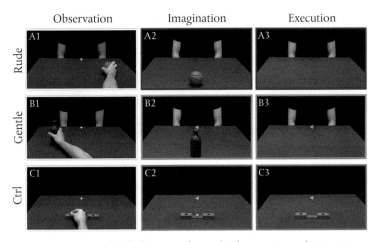

Fig. 4.2 Experimental task design. Left panel: Observation task. Participants observed a right hand moving an object rightwards (A1) or leftwards (B1). The observed action was performed gently or rudely and the task required the participants to focus on the style of the action. For the control condition, the participants observed the right hand placing a ball in the right-hand or left-hand box (C1). Middle panel: Imagination task. Participants had to imagine themselves passing an object to a person positioned in front of them, using either a gentle or a rude vitality form. In the central part of the screen a cue indicated the vitality forms (blue for gentle; red for rude) and the direction of the imagined action (A2, B2). For the control condition, participants had to imagine placing the ball in the box according to the direction of the cue (C2). Right panel: Execution task. The participants had to hold a package of crackers and move it with a rude (A3, red colour) or gentle (B3, blue colour) vitality form toward the person sitting in front of them. For the control condition, the participants had to place the small ball in the box (adapted from Di Cesare et al., 2015).

Speech vitality forms

As well as by gestures and actions, vitality forms can also be conveyed through speech. Depending on the attitude of the speaker towards the listener or their mood, the vitality form of their

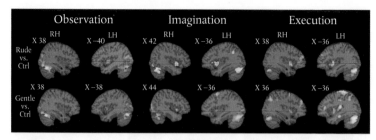

Fig. 4.3 Brain activations linked to vitality form processing. Parasagittal sections show the insular responses in the two hemispheres resulting from the contrast between the actions executed in a rude or gentle manner and actions executed without clear vitality forms in the three experimental conditions of observation, imagination, and execution.

Abbreviations: LH = left hemisphere, RH = right hemisphere (adapted from Di Cesare et al., 2015).

speech can vary; to continue using our previous example, it can be gentle or rude. The capacity to perceive speech vitality forms is already present in infants (Stern, 1985). Indeed, during mother–child interactions, the mother frequently pronounces words using characteristically childish language. Specifically, she adapts her language to the perceptive capacity of the child, appropriately slowing down her speech (Anderson & Jaffe, 1972; Malloch & Trevarthen, 2009).

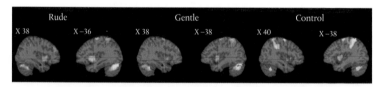

Fig. 4.4 Conjunction analysis on the activations of the insula in the three experimental conditions, observation, imagination, and execution, of actions executed rudely (left) or gently (centre) and the control activations (right) with actions executed without any clear vitality form (adapted from Di Cesare et al., 2015).

The question naturally arises as to whether the DCI, which is involved in the processing of action vitality forms, is also involved in encoding speech vitality forms. This has been addressed with an fMRI study (Di Cesare, Fasano, Errante et al., 2016), in which right-handed participants were presented with auditory stimuli consisting of four Italian action verbs ('*dammi*' [give], '*prendi*' [take], '*tocca*' [touch], and '*strappa*' [tear]) pronounced by an actor and an actress using two different vitality forms, rude and gentle (vitality form condition). The control condition consisted in listening to each verb in two conditions: the robot condition, in which the stimuli were produced by a robotic voice completely lacking in any form of vitality, and the scrambled condition, in which the components of the vitality forms were scrambled. In the robot condition, understanding the meaning of the action verbs was possible without the support of any vitality form, while in the scrambled condition the meanings and vitality forms of the verbal stimuli were fully opaque, with only their physical properties (pitch and amplitude) being preserved.

The results are shown in Fig. 4.5A. Listening to action verbs expressed with either a gentle or rude vitality form induced the activation of the superior temporal gyrus, left inferior parietal lobule, left premotor, left prefrontal cortex, and the posterior part of the inferior frontal gyrus and, most importantly, a bilateral activation of the DCI. A similar activation pattern was observed for the robot condition, with the sole exception of the insula, which activated only in the vitality form condition. Listening to the scrambled stimuli produced activation of the auditory temporal areas exclusively. The conjunction analysis of the contrast between the three conditions showed a clear activation of the left-hand DCI, which is

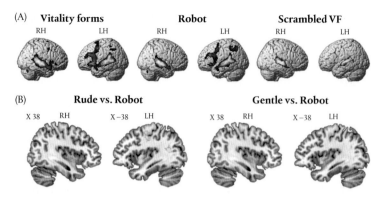

Fig. 4.5 (A) Brain activations obtained while listening to different stimuli categories. (B) Parasagittal sections showing the activations that resulted from contrasting a rude voice with a robotic voice and a gentle voice with a robotic voice (adapted from Di Cesare, Fasano, Errante et al., 2016).

Abbreviations: LH = left hemisphere, RH = right hemisphere.

specific for listening to verbs pronounced by a human voice with a given vitality form (Fig. 4.5B).

The finding that the DCI was activated when participants listened to action verbs cannot simply be accounted for by the meaning of those verbs. Indeed, it was activated only when participants listened to action verbs pronounced with a given vitality form, although the meaning conveyed by the robotic voice was exactly the same. The contrast between the vitality form condition and the scrambled condition clearly indicates that the DCI activation was related to the physical properties (intensity and frequency) of the human voice pronouncing the action verbs. Indeed in both conditions, the physical properties of the auditory stimuli were the same, but the DCI only activated in the vitality form condition.

Di Cesare and colleagues ran a further fMRI study to assess whether the DCI is activated not only by listening to action verbs with different vitality forms but also by imagining pronouncing those verbs in that manner (Di Cesare et al., 2018). Participants were asked to perform two tasks: a listening task and a speech imagination task. In the listening task, the participants were presented with three action verbs ['prendi' (take), 'tocca' (touch), 'chiudi' (close)] pronounced by two actors (a male and a female) in a gentle and a rude manner (vitality condition). As a control condition, the participants listened to the spelling of three nonsensical words (D-I-M-A, I-R-P-A, M-A-P-A) pronounced by the same actors. The actors pronounced the nonsensical words with the same physical properties of the vitality speech stimuli (pitch, amplitude) but did not convey any vitality form. In the speech imagination task, the participants were required to imagine pronouncing the same action verbs of the listening task in a rude or gentle way, or to imagine pronouncing the three nonsensical words.

The results showed that listening to action verbs pronounced with gentle or rude vitality forms produced an activation of the parieto-frontal circuit related to action understanding, stronger on the left side, together with a strong activation of the temporal superior frontal gyrus bilaterally. Imagining pronouncing the same action verbs with the same vitality forms produced a similar activation pattern, except for the superior temporal areas, and a stronger activation of the rostral prefrontal lobe. Fig. 4.6A shows the overlapping of areas activated in both tasks. Most importantly, the conjunction analysis showed that the DCI was activated in both tasks (Fig. 4.6B).

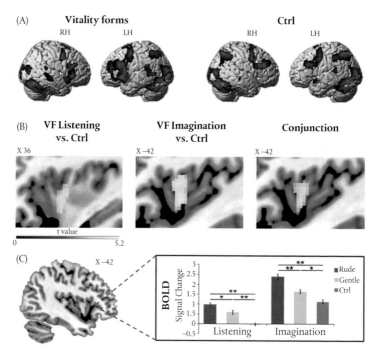

Fig. 4.6 Brain activations in speech processing. (A) Overlapping of areas active during the listening and imaging tasks obtained with a conjunction analysis for both vitality and control conditions. (B) Parasagittal sections showing the left insular activations during the speech session when contrasting the vitality and the control condition during the listening and imaging tasks. The conjunction analysis of the speech session revealed a common activation of the dorso-central sector of the insula in both tasks (A, right side). (C) BOLD signal changes extracted from the left DCI, resulting from the conjunction analysis of the speech tasks (listening, imaging). The horizontal line above the columns indicates the comparisons between the rude vitality form, the gentle vitality form, and the control (adapted from Di Cesare et al., 2018).

Anatomical and Functional Characteristics of the Dorso-Central Insula

The studies reviewed so far indicate that the DCI possesses the mirror property, selectively responding to our own and other people's vitality forms related to hand actions and speech. The finding that the DCI is involved in processing our own vitality forms and those of others, fits with the anatomical and functional characteristics of this portion of the insula in both non-human primates and humans.

We mentioned in Chapter 1 that electrical stimulation of the insular region of the monkey elicits a wide range of various motor responses, depending on which portion of the insula is being stimulated (p. 25). While the stimulation of the anterior insula mainly results in ingestive actions (dorsally) and in disgust reactions (ventrally), stimulation of the DCI elicits movements of body parts with a rich representation of those of the upper limbs (Caruana et al., 2011; Jezzini et al., 2012). A similar organization pattern has been reported by Florian Kurth and colleagues in humans (Kurth et al., 2010). In a meta-analysis based on a very large number of functional neuroimaging studies, these authors found four distinct functional fields in the human insula: the sensorimotor, the socio-emotional, the olfactory–gustatory, and the cognitive. The human sensorimotor field corresponds to the analogous sensorimotor functional field in the monkey. It also corresponds to the sector of the insula involved in vitality form processing.

Because this sector is not directly connected with the primary cortex (F1), the question arises as to how the DCI might modulate arm action and speech production. As emphasized in Chapter 2 (pp. 40–47) the role of the parieto-frontal network in representing and controlling hand and mouth actions is critical, therefore it could be surmised that the DCI controls the expression of hand action and speech vitality forms by modulating the activity of this network. Indeed, tract-tracing investigations in monkeys and a probabilistic tractography study in humans has shown that the DCI is connected with all three key nodes of the arm/hand control network: the inferior parietal lobule, the ventral premotor cortex, and prefrontal area 46 (Gerbella et al., 2011; Jezzini et al., 2015; Borra et al., 2017; Di Cesare et al., 2019). This is in line with further studies showing that the DCI is also connected with the portion of the second somatosensory cortex with hand and arm representation (Cipolloni & Pandya, 1999), as well as with the central part of the cingulate cortex (Pandya et al., 1981), in which electrical stimulation evokes arm movement in both monkeys and humans (Luppino et al., 1991; Picard & Strick, 1996).

As far as the visual and acoustic inputs are concerned, there is evidence that in humans the DCI is functionally connected with temporal structures encoding observed hand movements and the sounds of voices heard (Pernet et al., 2015). Similarly, studies on monkeys have found that the central part of the insula is connected with the anterior part of the superior temporal sulcus (Seltzer & Pandya, 1991), which as we have seen, hosts neurons responding to complex visual stimuli including different hand and arm movements (Perret et al., 1989), and with the rostral auditory parabelt (Mufson & Mesulam, 1982), which processes complex acoustic stimuli such as conspecific calls (Hackett, 2015).

Finally, it has been demonstrated that the DCI receives interoceptive information from a specific thalamic nucleus, the ventromedial posterior, that receives direct projections from lamina

I spinal neurons and hosts cells responding to many types of cutaneous stimuli such as pain, temperature, and affective touch (Craig, 2002, 2014). In addition, the DCI receives projections from sectors of the adjacent anterior and ventral insula that encode emotional and visceral states (Flynn, 1999), as well as from cortical regions integrating the emotional valence of sensory stimuli with reward and memory, such as the temporal pole and orbitofrontal and entorhinal cortices (Olson et al., 2007; Petrides, 2007) (Fig. 4.7).

Taken together, the functional and anatomical characteristics of the DCI reviewed here indicate that this portion of the insula plays a key role in integrating the information processed in the parieto-frontal network involved in controlling hand and mouth actions with the sensory, interoceptive, affective, and mnestic information sourcing from various cortical and subcortical structures. This explains how the DCI can modulate the execution of hand action as well as of speech according to the agent's affective

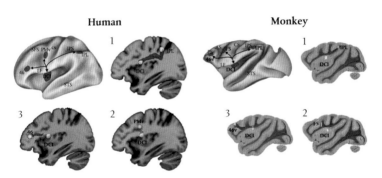

Fig. 4.7 Insular connections with the parieto-frontal grasping circuit in humans and monkeys. Overview of insular white matter tracts connecting the DCI with the parieto-frontal grasping circuit in humans (left side) and monkeys (left side). White matter tracts connecting the insula with the inferior parietal lobe (1), the premotor cortex (2) and the prefrontal area (3) (adapted from Di Cesare et al., 2019).

state, which can somehow be linked to memories of events and successes (or failures), the presence of some forms of motivation, or to the expectation of a reward or a potential threat, etc.

This also explains the kind of transformation that is involved in DCI mirror responses. The sensory representations evoked by seeing actions executed by others with one vitality form rather than another, e.g. gently rather than rudely, or hearing words spoken gently rather than roughly, are transformed in the DCI into the motor representations that give actions and speech that particular vitality form when we execute or produce them ourselves. Through this transformation, the sensory information relative to the actions we observe and the words we hear is processed by the same cortical and subcortical structures that are usually recruited to integrate our own affective and motivational states, memories, expectations, and so on, when we ourselves are acting or speaking with one particular vitality form rather than another (Fig. 4.8).

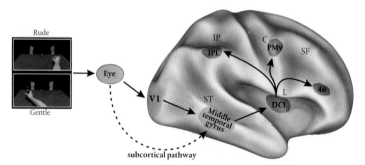

Fig. 4.8 The principal anatomical and cortical pathways by which the observation of an action executed with a given form of vitality reaches the same cortical centres that would be activated if the observer were to execute that action themselves with that kind of vitality form.

Abbreviations: V1 = primary visual cortex, ST = superior temporal sulcus, IP = intraparietal sulcus, C = central sulcus, SF = superior frontal sulcus, IPL = inferior parietal lobule, PMv = ventral premotor cortex, L = lateral scissure, DCI = dorso-central insula.

The Chapter in Brief

In this chapter, we have seen that mirror responses are not related exclusively to action goals and emotions. They also concern the dynamic forms that Daniel Stern called *vitality forms*, which characterize the unfolding of actions. A number of fMRI studies have shown that the DCI selectively responds to the execution, imagination and observation of hand actions and speech rendered with a given vitality form (e.g. rudely or gently). The anatomical and functional characteristics of the DCI corroborates the view that this portion of the insula plays a key role in processing our own hand action and speech vitality forms and those of others. The mirror responses of the DCI involve a transformation of the sensory representations relative to other people's actions and speech, into the motor representations that contribute to shaping the planning and execution of the observer's hand actions and speech and attributing them with a particular vitality form.

Research on the neural underpinnings of vitality forms is still in the very early stages and there is no doubt that much still remains to be done in order to fully understand how our own vitality forms and those of other people are processed. In this regard, it is worth noting that all the studies cited in the preceding pages focus on the characteristic modulation of vitality forms in the action domain and have attributed a distinctive role to the DCI in the representation of these forms, both when the actions were executed personally or observed while being executed by others. But what happens in the emotion domain?

In Stern's view, vitality forms identify actions as well as emotions. A bout of vomiting differs from a slight feeling of disgust, where the difference lies not just in the *content*, but also, and above all, in the *form* of the emotional reaction. Following this view, we might wonder whether there could be a cortical or subcortical structure (or a set of structures) deputed to modulate an emotional reaction such as disgust. And we might wonder whether something similar could hold true for the other emotional reactions. Should we expect to discover that the DCI is somehow involved in this modulation, independently of the kind of emotional reaction? Or could it be that this function involves other brain structures or networks?

Answering these and other related questions will be a challenge for future research, a challenge that will be critical as it should enable us to shed new light on the processes and representations involved in the basic forms of social interactions.

CHAPTER 5

MIRRORING
AND UNDERSTANDING

In the previous chapters we have examined mirror responses in the domains of action, emotion, and vitality forms. We have seen there are mirror responses that are selective for observed action goals, for facial expressions or bodily movements that are imbued with a particular emotional significance and for the manner in which an action is performed; we have also seen that these responses involve a mechanism of sensorimotor or visceromotor transformation. In these two final chapters we will take a step further, introducing and discussing the claim that the mirror mechanism can play a distinctive role in our understanding of other people's actions, emotions, and vitality forms. As without a doubt this is the most debated of all the issues we have tackled in this book, we have decided to devote this chapter entirely to a review of the data collected over the last twenty years that supports the claim. In the last chapter we will reflect on what kind of understanding, if any, can be triggered by the mirror mechanism and we will attempt to rebut the main objections raised against our proposal.

Mirroring Brains. Giacomo Rizzolatti and Corrado Sinigaglia, Oxford University Press. © Oxford University Press 2023. DOI: 10.1093/oso/9780198871705.003.0005

Action Observation and Execution

We will start with the action domain. In Chapter 2 we discussed and defended the claim that the mirror mechanism involves a transformation of the sensory representations concerning observed actions into motor representations similar to those which would occur if the observer themselves were planning and executing the same kind of actions (pp. 64–67). If this is in fact so, then it is to be expected that observing a particular action would have an effect on the execution of that same kind of action and vice versa.[1]

Wolfgang Prinz and colleagues at the Max Planck Institute for Psychological Research of Munich and later of the Max Planck

---

[1] We are certainly not the first to formulate such a hypothesis. Probably the primacy here is to be attributed to William James who maintained that the representation of an action to some extent 'awakens' its actual execution (1890). More recently, Anthony Greenwald (1970), followed by Wolfgang Prinz (1987, 1990), formulated what is now known as the ideomotor theory, hypothesizing that observing an action would evoke an image, similar to that of proximal and possibly distal sensory effects, that is involved in the planning and control of that action, so facilitating its execution. The greater the similarity of the two images, the greater will be the facilitation effect that observing the action will have on its execution. Thus, perception and action would share a common representational format, which would not only explain how observing an action can have an effect on its execution, but also why the execution of an action can have an impact on observing that action. There is no doubt that the ideomotor theory and the related idea of perception and action having a common code are very close to our hypothesis regarding the properties of mirror responses and the relative sensorimotor transformations. There are also points of difference, starting from the emphasis we place on the motor representation of action goal(s), rather than on the image of the proximal or distal sensory effects, both in producing and in observing the action. For a detailed analysis of the ideomotor approach, see also Hommel et al. (2001), Hommel (2013), and Stock and Stock (2004), among others, for a historical review.

Institute for Human Cognitive and Brain Sciences of Leipzig, conducted an elegant series of behavioural experiments, demonstrating that the presentation of stimuli showing very simple actions, such as raising the index or the middle fingers, facilitates the observer's motor response when they are asked to execute an action congruent with that shown in the stimulus, even when that action is not relevant to the task. In one of their studies, the authors required their participants to watch a five-frame video of an animated hand resting on a flat surface with numbers identifying the fingers to be raised (Brass et al., 2000). The paradigm consisted of two blocks; in the first, the participants were asked to reproduce the action seen on the video as quickly as possible, raising their index or middle fingers according to the stimulus shown. In the second block, in which the index finger was indicated as 1 and the middle finger as 2, they were asked to raise the finger corresponding to the number stimulus shown (the symbolic cue condition) as quickly as possible. In both blocks, the number and the finger raised in the video were congruent in half of the trials, e.g. the number 1 appeared while the index finger was being raised; in the other half, the number 1 appeared when the middle finger was being raised (see Fig. 5.1 top). In general, the participants were quicker in raising their fingers when their response depended on the action they observed than when their response depended on the number stimulus. Moreover, the crucial point was that the participants were significantly quicker when the number indicating the finger was congruent with the finger that was actually raised in the video (Fig. 5.1 bottom), in spite of the fact that the congruence was not relevant to the task, which

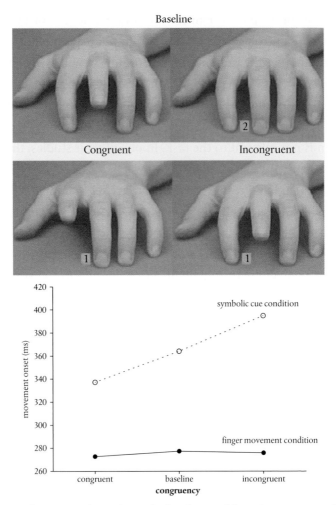

Fig. 5.1 The picture above shows the last frame of the video sequence of the Baseline, Congruent and Incongruent trials. In the Baseline trial, the finger to be raised was shown directly or indicated by a symbolic cue (numbers 1 or 2). The stimuli were identical for both conditions in the Congruent and Incongruent trials. The chart below shows the movement onset (RT) as a function of congruency (Congruent, Baseline, and Incongruent) and condition (finger movement, symbolic cue). In the symbolic cue condition, the observed finger movement was irrelevant to the execution of the task; similarly, it was irrelevant when the task consisted in moving the congruent or incongruent finger (adapted from Brass et al., 2000).

simply required the participants to concentrate on the number indicating the finger to be raised.[2]

Marcello Costantini and colleagues at the Chieti and Rome Universities showed that a similar facilitation effect could not be reducible to those cases where an observed action and an executed action involve the same movements, but it can be induced when the congruence concerns the goals of the observed action and of the actually executed action (Costantini et al., 2008). The authors designed a series of behavioural studies to systematically explore which aspects of an observed action could have a priming motor effect. The participants were shown a rapid sequence of images depicting meaningless or meaningful actions. The results showed that the participants responded more rapidly when the images showed actions with the same goal, even when it was attained by different means or different effectors. For example, the

---

[2] In a later study, Prinz et al. modified the paradigm; the participants were asked to raise or lower their index fingers as soon as the corresponding movement appeared in the video and their reaction times were compared. The results showed that the participants were quicker in raising or lowering their index finger when the action was congruent with that shown in the video (Brass et al., 2001). The congruence effect remained, although somewhat reduced, when the action in the video was shown upside down. In fact, here too, the participants were quicker in responding when the required action was congruent with the action seen in the video. A later study by Roman Liepelt et al. (Liepelt et al., 2009), adopted the same paradigm as Brass et al. (2000), with the difference that in one-third of the trials the index finger and the middle finger in the video were clamped to the table, and in another third, the thumb and the ring finger were blocked. The participants were significantly slower in raising the index and middle fingers in the trials in which the corresponding fingers in the video were immobilized, in spite of the fact that they had been told specifically to concentrate exclusively on the number that would appear on the hand and ignore anything else. By recording the EEG signal from the participants' scalps, these authors found that when the finger movement occurred in response to the picture showing a hand with the index and middle fingers clamped to the table, the slowing of response times was reflected in a decrease of the lateralized readiness potentials (LRP) that represent a component of the EEG signal, typically used as a temporal marker of motor preparation (Liepelt et al., 2009).

sight of a person flattening a box with a foot facilitated the action of flattening for the participants even when executed with a different effector (a hand instead of a foot) and with a different target object (a tin instead of a box).

Our hypothesis does not imply that the effect exerted by the observed action on the executed action has to be facilitatory. Quite the opposite: if the observed action evokes a motor representation of an action goal that is in some way at odds with the action that the observer is preparing to execute, it is likely that it will constitute an impediment to that action. This is something you can try at home for yourself; move your right arm so as to draw an imaginary vertical or horizontal line in the air. When you have perfected the movement to the point at which your arm movements are regular, and the imaginary lines are of the same length, try to imagine continuing to draw those lines while watching another person, or a robotic arm, doing likewise. You may not be aware of this, but observing someone else executing a different movement to the one you yourself are executing interferes with your own execution of the line, as James Kilner and colleagues demonstrated with an elegant behavioural study (Kilner et al., 2003). As in our thought experiment, their participants were asked to draw vertical or horizontal lines while observing another human being or a robotic arm making the same or qualitatively different movements. They found that when observed movements were not congruent, they interfered significantly with the participants' performance. However, the most interesting finding was that the interference effect was absent when the participants were observing movements made by a robotic arm (Fig. 5.2).[3]

[3] Ulrich Drost et al. of the Max Planck Institutes in Munich and Leipzig found similar interference effects in a study they designed involving expert pianists and

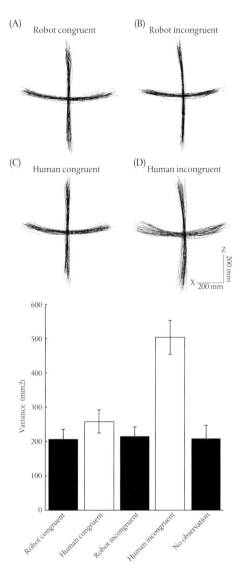

Fig. 5.2 The image above shows the horizontal and vertical movements made by the subject while observing the robot making congruent (A) and incongruent movements (B), and while observing the experimenter making congruent (C) and incongruent movements (D). The chart below shows the analysis of the variances of the movements in the five conditions (A–D plus a baseline condition with no observation). The only condition that differed significantly from the baseline movement condition was that in which the subjects watched the experimenter making arm movements that were incongruent with the movements they were supposed to be making themselves (adapted from Kilner et al., 2003).

The aim of these studies was to explore the effect that *observing* an action would have on executing a similar or incongruent action. However, our hypothesis also implies that the *execution* of an action can facilitate or interfere with the observation of that action or of a similar action. A study of particular relevance to this, consisting of combining the preparation, observation, and execution of an action, was conducted by Laila Craighero and colleagues at the Universities of Parma and Ferrara (Craighero et al., 2002). Their participants were instructed to prepare to grasp a bar placed at a 45-degree angle between their thumb and index finger, and then to proceed with the actual grasping with their right hand as soon as they were presented with a visual stimulus. The stimulus consisted of a mirror image of the right hand, depicted as if in the final configuration for grasping the bar oriented either clockwise or anticlockwise. It emerged that their participants' reaction times were faster when there was a similarity between the hand position as depicted in the triggering visual stimulus and the final position of the grasping hand, the fastest responses being those where this similarity was closest. As the authors themselves pointed out, the difference in reaction times could be explained as the facilitation

---

guitarists. The authors asked their participants to play a chord in response to a visual stimulus of musical notes accompanied by a sound effect produced by another instrument (piano, organ, guitar, flute, or voice), which could either be congruous or incongruous with the chord the participants had been asked to play. Although the sound effect was totally irrelevant to the task, the pianists were slower in playing the chord indicated by the visual stimulus when the sound effect was incongruent and produced with a keyboard (piano or organ); the interference effect disappeared when the incongruent sound was associated with other instruments. Similarly, the guitar players were slower in playing the assigned chord only when the incongruent sound effect was produced with a guitar. According to the authors, the interference effect can be attributed to the transformation of the sound representations into their corresponding motor representations which, obviously, are different for pianists and guitar players (Drost et al., 2007).

effect of the motor preparation on processing the congruent visual stimulus as well as the similarity between the motor representations of the observed and the executed actions.

Chris Miall and colleagues at the University of Birmingham designed an oddball paradigm to evaluate whether the motor representation of an action can influence its visual representation. They set their participants a visual discrimination task, which consisted of identifying a target image (a hand with the index and middle fingers spread out in the classic V for victory sign, or with the index finger and thumb touching to form the universal OK sign), intercalated in a sequence of images showing a hand with fingers spread out or rotating on itself, presented either in a predictable or a random sequence (Miall et al., 2006). The participants were asked to pronounce a syllable as soon as they individuated the target image. While doing this, they were asked to spread their fingers or rotate their hand in a movement that was congruent or incongruent with the sequence of the movements shown. The results indicated that the participants were quicker in replying not only when the image sequence was predictable but also, and above all, when it represented an action that was congruent with that which they were executing. The predictability of the image sequence alone did not have any effect on the discrimination task when the images represented an action that was incongruent with the action the participants were executing.[4]

---

[4] Marta Bortoletto et al. conducted an EEG study which showed that the motor priming of an action can modulate its perceptive processing in the first 200 ms after stimulus presentation (Bortoletto et al., 2011). By analysing the visual ERPs, the authors found a significant alteration of two components (VPP and N170) that are considered to reflect high-level processing of visual information relating to various parts of the body. This would indicate that motor representations evoked in preparation of the action would have a direct effect not only on its execution but

Taken together, these studies show that an observed action and an executed action may be intrinsically linked, sharing a neural substrate and a representational format that would allow the observation of an action to have a specific impact on its execution to the same extent that the planning and executing of an action would significantly influence the observation of an action being executed by someone else. The functional characteristics of mirror responses as identified in Chapter 2 and the kind of sensorimotor transformation that they trigger, seem to offer a natural explanation for both these effects. In fact, on the one hand, when we observe an action we recruit, albeit partially, the same processes and motor representations that would be recruited if we ourselves were to perform the observed action. This would explain both the facilitation effect that occurs when the observer is asked to execute a task congruent with the task being observed, and the interference effect that has been found when the observer has to execute an action that is significantly different from that being observed. On the other hand, the motor processes and representations recruited while observing a given action are involved in processing the sensory information regarding this action, which explains why action preparation and execution may affect perceptual discrimination.[5]

---

also on the processing of sensory representations, visual in this case, concerning the action being observed.

[5] It should be mentioned here that motor priming effects can be attributed also to the sensorimotor transformations induced by the responses of canonical neurons to the observation of objects, regardless of whether they are effective or potential action targets. Several studies have shown how the sight of an object can facilitate the production of a congruent action (Craighero et al., 1999, 2002; Witt et al., 2005; Witt & Profitt, 2008), even when the representation of the object is not in itself relevant to executing the action (Tucker & Ellis, 1998, 2001, 2004; Ellis & Tucker, 2000; Costantini et al., 2010).

Observing and Understanding Actions

So far, we have only considered the implications of the sensori-motor transformations that are typically triggered by mirror responses regarding the facilitation or interference effects relative to the observation or execution of an action. However, according to our claim, not only do the sensorimotor transformations typical of mirror responses involve these effects, they also (and above all) play a distinctive role in understanding the action being observed. In other words, if observing an action triggers recruitment of the same motor processes and representations that would have been recruited had the observer been planning the action and executing it themselves, then it also enables the observer to understand the observed action and to individuate its possible goals.[6]

Is there evidence to support this claim? Most definitely. In the following sections we will show that there are at least *four* lines of evidence to suggest that the sensorimotor transformations typical of mirror responses play a distinctive role in understanding actions executed by others.

Action and perceptual judgement

The first line of evidence calls on a series of studies aimed at system-atically investigating how motor processes and representations can

---

[6] This does not mean to say that the understanding of an action linked to the sensorimotor transformations typical of mirror responses does not imply a facilitation/interference in action execution and vice versa. We simply wish to point out that mirror responses and the sensorimotor transformations involved can play a role in understanding an action being observed, without that action having to be physically executed. See also Beets et al. (2010).

have an effect on the way in which people judge what they observe. The logic behind these studies is similar to that of the research we have mentioned earlier, though of course the dependent variable is different. If it is true that observing an action elicits a mirror response and that this response plays a role in understanding that action, it is to be expected that the execution of an action similar to that being observed will affect the observer's perceptual judgement. In fact, the execution of that action would recruit the same motor processes and representations that are evoked when the action is observed.

An example will help to make this clearer. Imagine that you are standing on a moving walkway that has been turned off and right in front of you there is a video of two people walking. Let's call them Peter and John. Your task is to figure out whether Peter is walking more quickly than John. Unless they are walking very fast, the task should not be particularly difficult, even if the difference in speed is minimal.[7] But what happens if the moving walkway is set in motion again and you yourself start walking? You would soon realize that your walking would have an impact on how you judge Peter and John's relative speed; at least, this is what Alissa Jacobs and Maggie Shiffrar of Rutgers University found in an elegant experiment conducted some years ago (Jacobs and Shiffrar, 2005).

In their experiment, Jacobs and Shiffrar used Gunnar Johansson's *point-light walker display technique* in which a person is filmed while walking in the dark, but the visible action is reduced to a limited number of luminous markers attached to their head and joints

---

[7] According to Weber's Law, the ability to perceive the difference between two stimuli is inversely proportional to the physical intensity of the original stimulus. In the present case, this means that the quicker Peter and John walk, the less able are we to pick up the slighter differences in their relative speed.

(Johansson, 1973). As action presented in this way is easily identifiable (among others, see also Blake and Shiffrar, 2007 for a review), Jacobs and Shiffrar asked their participants to evaluate the relative speed of two individuals walking side by side at speeds between 2 km and 6 km per hour, with a constant difference between their speeds of 0.5 km per hour. The participants were asked to judge which of the two individuals was the faster, while engaged in three conditions: standing still on a moving walkway, walking on a moving walkway, and cycling on a cyclette. As expected, walking impacted on how the participants judged the relative speeds of the two individuals. In fact, when they were walking, their judgement was less accurate than when they were standing still. It is interesting to note that this effect was not present when the participants were pedalling on the cyclette, meaning that it cannot be attributed simply to the fact that the participants were doing two different things at the same time (moving and judging), but was due rather to the fact that the action executed and the action judged recruited the same motor processes and representations.[8]

Antonia Hamilton and colleagues at University College London conducted a series of similar behavioural and brain imaging experiments. In one study, participants were shown a video in which

---

[8] In a similar vein, Andreas Wohlschläger of the Max Planck Institute in Monaco ran a study in which the participants were shown a set of discs arranged to form an ambiguously rotating imaginary circle; while turning a handle without being able to see their hand, they were asked to judge whether the discs were moving clockwise or anticlockwise. Wohlschläger found that the participants' judgement was influenced by the kind of action they were executing; when they were turning the handle clockwise, they tended to see the circumference of the discs move in the same direction, and vice versa. He found the same effect in a later study in which the participants were asked simply to imagine turning the handle, hence just planning the action without physically executing it (Wohlschläger, 2001).

a person lifted a box with one hand and placed it on a shelf. Their task was to estimate the weight of the box, which could be one of five weights: 50, 250, 450, 650, or 850 grams (Hamilton et al., 2004). As in Jacobs and Shiffrar's experiment, the participants were asked to formulate their estimate in three conditions: *active*, in which they themselves lifted a box that was either light (150 gr) or heavy (750 gr); *passive*, in which they simply held one of the two boxes in their hand without lifting it; *neutral*, in which their activity was limited to watching the video. The participants showed a clear predisposition to underestimate the weight of the box that was being lifted in the video when they themselves were holding the heavier box, while they overestimated its weight when they were holding the lighter box. This predisposition was much more noticeable, to the extent that it doubled, in the active condition when participants had to lift (and not simply to hold) the box themselves.

In another study using an fMRI scanner, Hamilton and colleagues set their participants the same task in the active and neutral conditions (Hamilton et al., 2006). The BOLD signal showed a robust correlation between the over- and underestimation of the weight of the box and the activation of a network of cortical areas including a portion of the inferior frontal gyrus, part of the primary motor cortex of the central sulcus that controls hand movements, and a small region of the inferior intraparietal sulcus. As these are motor areas with the mirror property, this shows that the motor processes and representations evoked while observing an action can affect the ability of the observer to make estimations or judgements.[9]

---

[9] In a repetitive transcranial magnetic stimulation (rTMS) study, Hamilton et al. stimulated the inferior frontal gyrus with a train of magnetic impulses; the inferior frontal gyrus in fact is one of the key nodes of the parieto-frontal network, whose

The research discussed so far shows how the contribution to perceptual judgement of the motor representations evoked while observing an action can relate to certain physical properties of that action (e.g. the speed at which it is being executed) or of the object involved (the weight). However, this alone does not tell us if and how the mirror responses and consequent sensorimotor transformations can contribute directly to understanding the action, to identifying its potential goals, and to realizing which of these is/are the goal(s) of the action. Of course, the motor representation contribution in all these studies is *content-specific*, in the sense that the effect on the perceptual judgement depends on the kind of goal and action represented motorically; the motor representation of walking (but not of pedalling!) contributed significantly to the perceptual judgement of the relative speed of the observed action. The same was true for the motor representation of lifting in relation to estimating the weight of an object being

mirror activity correlated with the over- and underestimating weight effect (Pobric & Hamilton, 2006). As in the preceding studies, the participants were asked to estimate the weight of a box that they saw being lifted with one hand and placed on a shelf. There were two control conditions: in the first, there was a change of scene (instead of a box being lifted, the participants were shown a film of a bouncing ball), but the task was the same, i.e. to estimate the weight of the object, while in the second the scene was that of the box being lifted with one hand and placed on the shelf, but the participants were asked to estimate how long the hand remained visible. The authors found that applying the rTMS to the inferior frontal gyrus had a negative effect on the accuracy of the estimation of the weight of the box. Of particular interest was the fact that this effect was only present when the participants were asked to estimate the weight of the box that was being lifted and moved. There was no such effect when they were asked to estimate the weight of the bouncing ball nor when they were asked to estimate the length of time the hand was visible on the screen. This is further evidence that sensorimotor transformations typical of mirror responses play a distinctive role in judging an observed action. Not only do they correlate with the over- and underestimation effect, but if impeded they significantly reduce the accuracy of perceptual judgement.

lifted by someone else. And there is no doubt that identifying certain physical properties of the action being observed or the object
involved in the action can contribute to the understanding of that
action. But is this the full extent of the contribution that mirror
responses can provide to understanding actions? According to
our claim, the distinctive role played by mirror responses when
observing actions depends above all on the fact that the sensorimotor transformations they implicate contribute to identifying
the action goal. But do we really have evidence that this is in fact
the case? In other words, do we have evidence that the motor
representations evoked while observing an action influence the
perceptual judgement when this relates not only to physical
properties such as speed and weight, but also, and above all, to
the goal(s) of the observed action?

Convincing evidence in this direction comes from an elegant study conducted by Luigi Cattaneo and colleagues at the
Universities of Trento, Grenoble, and Arizona. The study used a
visuo-motor adaptation paradigm coupled with transcranial magnetic stimulation (TMS) (Cattaneo et al., 2011). The objective was to
see if (and if, how) the repeated execution of an action determines
adaptation when the action is observed rather than being executed, inducing an after-effect on the corresponding perceptual
judgement. In the first experiment, a spherical bowl containing
dried chickpeas was placed to the right of the participants, who
were instructed to push the chickpeas away or pull them closer
on the appearance of a visual stimulus which remained visible for
approximately 60 seconds. An opaque screen was placed above
their arm to block their vision of what their hand was doing. Once
the motor adaptation task was completed, the participants were
shown visual stimuli depicting a hand touching a ball at various

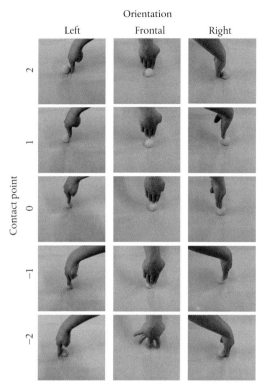

Fig. 5.3 Visual stimuli employed in the two experiments. The full set of hand stimuli in the three different orientations and five different contact points with the ball is shown (adapted from Cattaneo et al., 2011).

contact points; the task consisted in identifying the goal of the observed action.

The illustrations in Fig. 5.3 will help to make this clearer. Imagine that you have been asked to decide whether the hand in the pictures is pushing the ball away or pulling it closer. It is reasonable to suppose that your reply will vary according to the position of the point of contact between the hand and the ball, so it is very likely that you will have little doubt that in the images in the squares at the top (contact point + 2), the goal is to push the ball away, whereas in the squares at the bottom (contact point −2), the goal is to pull it closer. You might be a little less certain when the contact points are at +1 and −1, but if pressed for an answer, you will probably feel justified in saying that the hand is pushing the ball away or drawing it closer, respectively. But what about contact point 0, when the hand is perpendicular to the ball, and the contact point is in the direct centre? The contact point offers no information about the possible outcome of the action, so you would just have to guess.

This in fact was how the participants responded before the motor adaptation task, but what is particularly interesting is how they responded after the task (see Fig 5.3). After having spent 60 seconds repeatedly pulling the chickpeas closer, the participants showed a significant bias when judging the most ambiguous condition (contact point 0), deciding that the hand is pushing the ball away; vice versa, after 60 seconds repeatedly pushing the chickpeas away, the bias was to judge the action goal at contact 0 as pulling the ball closer. In both cases the stimulus was the same, but the way the participants judged it changed, with the change depending on the kind of motor adaptation, or in other words, by which motor representations they were adapted. If the adaptation involved the motor representation of pushing away, the after-effect on the perceptual judgement was a bias to respond that the goal was to pull the ball closer; on the contrary, if the adaptation involved the motor representation of pulling closer, the after-effect on the perceptual judgement was a bias to respond that the goal was to push the ball away.[10]

---

[10] Perceptual after-effects induced by motor adaptation have also been found in other studies, see for example, Müsseler and Hommel (1997), Müsseler et al. (2001), Nishimura and Yokosawa (2010). As in Cattaneo et al.'s study, in all these experiments the perceptual after-effects are due primarily to congruence

As the effect went from motor to visual and depended on how the action goal was represented motorically, it was more than justifiable to assume that it could be attributed mainly to the type of sensorimotor transformations that are characteristic of mirror responses. Cattaneo and colleagues carried out a second experiment to see if this was in fact the case. The adaptation task was identical to the first experiment. A single TMS pulse was delivered to the participants' ventral premotor cortex (PMv) as soon as they were shown the visual stimulus representing the action to be judged. The use of this protocol was based on the hypothesis that the effects of the TMS depend on the state of activation of the neural population being stimulated.

As we saw in Chapters 1 and 2, the PMv is not only an area where action goals such as grasping, pushing, etc. are motorically represented, but is also known to have the mirror property regarding action goals of this kind (see pp. 53–56). If it is true that the effect of the repeated execution of an action on perceptual judgement vis-à-vis the goal of an observed action is primarily due to the mirror mechanism, it would follow that stimulation of the PMv's activation state would interfere with the effect that the execution of the action has on perceptual judgement (Fig. 5.4).

More precisely, the expectation was that the participants would no longer tend to attribute the action they were observing with a goal diametrically opposed to the action they had repeatedly executed. And this, indeed, was what Cattaneo and colleagues found. In the trials during which the PMv was stimulated, their

between the motorically represented goals of the actions to be executed and the perceptual stimuli. However, unlike Cattaneo et al.'s study, the stimuli used in these experiments were mainly arrows or other symbols, more or less congruently oriented vis-à-vis the actions to be executed.

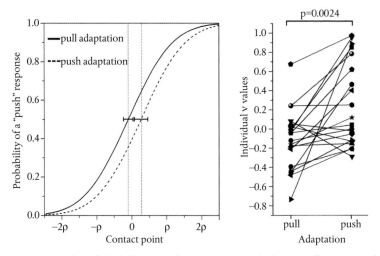

Fig. 5.4 Results of the behavioural experiment with the overall average of all the individual psychometric functions in the two motor adaptation conditions. A shift of the psychometric curve towards the left indicates an increased probability of categorizing the stimulus as 'push'. Vice-versa a shift to the right indicates a bias in favour of 'pull' responses (adapted from Cattaneo et al., 2011).

participants did in fact tend to reply randomly when presented with the image in which the point of contact of the hand with the ball gave no indication as to the possible action goal. However, that was not the case when the PMv was stimulated with a sham TMS, or if the stimulation was applied to a different cortical region, such as the primary motor cortex (Fig. 5.5).

Taken together, these studies provide sound evidence to support the claim that the mirror mechanism plays a distinctive role not only in facilitating execution of the observed action but also, and above all, in its relative perceptual judgement. This is the case both when the judgement regards the physical properties of the action and when it directly involves its apparent goal(s). Another

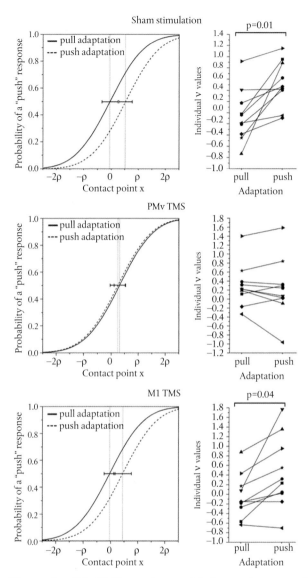

Fig. 5.5 The results of the TMS experiment with the grand-average of all the individual psychometric functions in the two motor adaptation conditions. As in the previous diagram, a shift of the psychometric curve towards the left indicates an increased probability of categorizing the stimulus as 'push'. Vice-versa, a shift to the right indicates a bias in favour of 'pull' responses. Note that the bias in the perceptual judgement was absent only when the PMv was stimulated. (adapted from Cattaneo et al., 2011).

important aspect is that the effect of the motor representations evoked by the mirror responses on perceptual judgement is *content-specific*, in that its content can vary with changes in the content of the representations. Think for a moment about walking, lifting, or moving chickpeas as in the last experiment we examined. In all these cases, repeated action modified the state of the observers' motor system, as it continuously recruited motor representations that would shortly have been recruited by observing a similar kind of action; this induced a sort of bias at perceptual level that caused the participants to modify their judgement of the observed action, even to the extent of changing their opinion about the action goal, as in Cattaneo et al.'s experiment (2011).

The contribution of motor expertise

A series of studies investigated the contribution of motor expertise to understanding observed actions and predicting the final outcome and possible related effects. These studies provide a second line of evidence that further corroborates the notion that mirror responses can have an effect on the observer's judgement and that this judgement can be linked to the degree of congruence between the observed and the motorically represented action.

In Chapter 2 (pp. 70–72), we mentioned the studies conducted by Calvo-Merino and colleagues (Calvo-Merino et al., 2005, 2006) and Cross and colleagues (Cross et al., 2006), which showed how mirror responses vary with the different levels of the observers' motor expertise. The greater an observer's expertise in a given action, the stronger and more selective were the mirror responses in the areas typically involved in the planning and execution of that kind of action. If mirror responses do play a distinctive role in understanding observed actions, and if they do in fact vary according to the level of the observer's motor expertise, it is to be expected that said level of motor expertise will have an influence on the understanding of the observed action, and will affect the reliability of the prediction of its outcome and possible consequences.

A number of studies carried out some years ago with the aim of exploring if and how motor processes and representations can influence the content of a given perceptual judgement provided some evidence of this. For instance, Bruno Repp and Günther Knoblich investigated acoustic perception by taking advantage of the so-called Tritone Paradox (Repp & Knoblich, 2007). This paradox consists in a sequentially played pair of tones separated by an interval of a half octave (a tritone), which some people perceive as ascending and others as descending. Repp and Knoblich asked a group of volunteers to judge the pitch change between twelve pairs of tones separated by a tritone just after pressing two keys on a computer keyboard with their forefinger, from left to right or right to left. The group was composed of expert pianists and randomly selected undergraduates; the tone pairs were randomly associated with the left-right and right-left sequences. The researchers found that while pressing the keys from left to right or right to left did not impact the control group's judgement regarding the pitch of the tone pairs, the expert pianists tended to judge the tone pair as ascending more often when they were pressing the keys from left to right than when they were pressing them from right to left. As all the participants executed the same actions, it is fair to assume that this effect depends primarily on the degree of expertise, in other words on the difference in their ability to represent the action motorically and anticipate its possible consequences.

A finding from a later study by Repp and Knoblich is even more interesting for our purposes (Repp & Knoblich, 2009). They investigated whether motor expertise can have an effect on acoustic perception when the action is *observed* instead of being *executed*. The paradigm was similar to that of the preceding experiment, but the authors added another condition in which the participants watched the experimenter pressing keys on a keyboard from left to right or right to left with their index finger. As in the preceding experiment, even though the action was always the same, only the pianists were affected by observing the experimenter, judging the tone pair as ascending more frequently when the experimenter pressed the keys from left to right.

Now the question is, can motor expertise influence the judgement of the observer even when this is concerned with the potential goals rather than the effects of the observed action? As we pointed out earlier, simply observing movements of luminous markers attached to major joints, as in point-light displays, is sufficient to facilitate identification of the represented action. However, this can depend on motor or visual expertise or even both. For example, we know that we tend to rely on our motor expertise when judging another person's gait. Indeed, we have difficulty with this kind of task if the visual stimuli seem to violate biomechanical constraints (as would be the case if the movement of the luminous markers were to be manipulated to represent walking backwards). If, on the other hand, we have to identify the person we see walking, visual expertise takes on a much more important role (Jacobs et al., 2004). But what happens if we have to identify the goal of the action we are observing? And how do we distinguish the effect that motor expertise can have on our ability to judge the observed action from the effect produced by visual expertise?

Antonino Casile and Martin Giese of the University of Tübingen used a motor training paradigm to supply an answer to these questions (Casile & Giese, 2006). The study was structured as three tests, in the first of which, a visual pre-test, the participants were consecutively shown two short point-light frames, in which ten luminous markers represented a person walking. The frames presented two identical gaits or two gaits with a minimal phase difference between the upper and lower limbs. The participants were asked to judge whether the observed gaits were identical or different. It is well known that human gait patterns are usually characterized by a phase difference of approximately 180 degrees between the two arms and the two legs. Casile and Giese manipulated this phase difference in order to create three prototypical point-light walkers, corresponding to phase differences of 180, 225, and 270 degrees (Fig. 5.6).

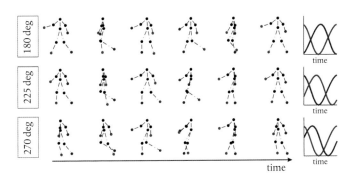

Fig. 5.6 The top row shows successive frames of a point-light walker with a 180-degree phase difference, corresponding to normal walking. The two rows below illustrate the prototype stimuli that were generated by manipulation of the phase difference between contralateral limbs (middle row, 225 degrees; bottom row, 270 degrees). The panels on the right show the horizontal components of the trajectories of the two hands in the three phases (adapted from Casile and Giese, 2006).

As was to be expected, the participants showed greater accuracy in identifying the gait pattern of the observed point-light walkers when the phase difference between the contralateral limbs was 180 degrees than when it was 225 degrees. The phase difference of 270 degrees produced the least accurate performance. However, this changed after the participants were given a brief motor training during which they were blindfolded and taught how to walk with a phase difference of 270 degrees. Although they had no visual feedback during the motor training phase, the participants' performance on the action identification task improved significantly when they were asked to judge the gait of point-light walkers when the phase difference was 270 degrees. There was no improvement when the phase difference was 180 and 225 degrees (Fig. 5.7).

The most interesting aspect was that the improvement in the performance on the identification task correlated directly with the

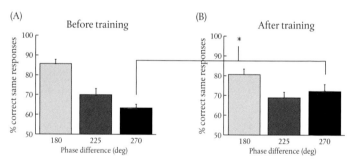

Fig. 5.7 The two panels show the percentages of correct action identification responses in trials in which the two stimuli had the same phase difference for the three prototypes (180, 225, and 270 degrees). (A) shows performances before motor training, (B) shows performance after motor training. The participants showed a significant improvement in the observed action identification task after the motor training, but only for the type of gait for which they had been trained (phase difference 270 degrees) even if the training did not include visual feedback (adapted from Casile, Giese, 2006).

level of motor training, as evidenced by the notable fluidity and low variability in the 270-degree phase difference gait. In other words, the better the participants were at executing the gait to be learnt, the better they were at identifying that type of gait when they saw it being performed by others, even without being able to count on a greater visual expertise.[11]

The idea that the observer can represent the observed action not only in visual, or more generally, in sensory terms, but also in motor terms by recruiting the same processes and representations they would use if they were to execute the action themselves, implies that motor expertise, as well as facilitating identification of the action goal, can significantly influence the ability to predict how the action will develop and in particular, whether it will achieve its goal.

Imagine you are watching television: your favourite basketball team is playing in the finals of the Euro league. Time is almost up, there is just one second of play to go and your team is one point behind. Your best shooter moves towards the free throw circle for two free throws. The first goes into the hoop and through the basket. During the second throw, at the very second that the ball leaves his hand and starts its trajectory towards the basket, by a quirk of fate there is a blackout. Your screen goes blank. You have no way of knowing whether the ball will actually go into the hoop and through the basket. There are two commentators, a journalist who has never played basketball but who has been present

---

[11] The study conducted by Heiko Hecht et al. provides further evidence on the impact of motor expertise on perceptual judgement. In this study, the authors found that after their participants had practised a two-arm circular movement blindfold, the accuracy of their perceptual judgement improved significantly when the action was observed rather than executed.

at thousands of games, and a former basketball champion who has played in thousands of games but for whom this is the first experience as commentator. When the lights go out, both make a prediction as to the outcome of the game. Let's suppose they make different predictions: Who would you trust more? You would probably put your money on the former champion and according to a study conducted by Salvatore Aglioti and colleagues at Rome's La Sapienza University and the University of Verona (Aglioti et al., 2008), you would have made the right decision.

Their participants were sports journalists and coaches with extensive visual but no practical experience (the expert watchers), former elite basketball players (the experts with extensive motor experience) and people with no basketball experience whatsoever (the novice group). They were asked to watch videoclips of players shooting free throws. The videos had ten different durations. For instance, they could be blocked after approximately 400–500 ms, when the players were loading the shot; after approximately 700–800 ms when the shooters' hands released the ball and it started its trajectory upwards to the hoop; after approximately 1200 ms when the ball started its downwards trajectory towards the hoop (Fig. 5.8).

After each viewing the participants were asked if, in their view, the ball would enter the hoop or not. If they were not sure of the answer, they replied 'I don't know'. The results show that generally, compared to the journalists, coaches, and novices, the elite players were quicker and more accurate in predicting the outcome of the action. The performance of the journalists and coaches did not differ in accuracy from that of the novices. It is interesting to note that the difference in accuracy between the elite players and the other two groups depended mostly on their ability to predict the outcome of the action during the first 710 ms, in which the

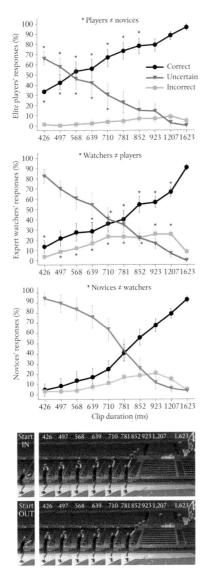

Fig. 5.8 Percentages of uncertain, correct, and incorrect responses made by the elite players, expert watchers, and novice groups at the different clip durations. The point of intersection between uncertain and correct response curves represents the clip duration at which correct responses were higher than uncertain responses. This occurred after 568 ms for elite athletes, after 710 ms for expert watchers and after 781 ms for novices (adapted from Aglioti et al., 2008).

crucial information was motor in nature and concerned the action of thrusting the ball. In addition, on examination of the uncertain responses it is clear that the novices only started to predict the outcome when the videos began to show the trajectory of the ball, while the uncertain responses of all three groups gradually decreased with the longer clips, which would seem to indicate that they used the same criteria to predict the outcome of the action. Notwithstanding this, the difference between the groups in terms of accuracy was significant, once again confirming that motor expertise counts more than visual expertise in the ability to forecast the outcome of the observed action.

Another interesting result came from a second experiment conducted by Aglioti and colleagues. They used single-pulse TMS to stimulate the primary motor cortex of their three groups of participants while they were watching three video clips of different lengths (568, 781, and 1,207 ms): the first two clips showed a basketball player shooting a ball at the basket in a free throw and the third showed a soccer player kicking a ball towards the goal. Although just watching the basketball player clips evoked an increase of the motor evoked potentials recorded from the abductor *digiti minimi* (the muscle in the small finger that is generally used in controlling the ball during a free throw) in all three groups, only the group of the elite players showed a significant modulation related to the outcome of the action (ball in/ball out). What was even more interesting was that this modulation occurred when the TMS pulse was delivered at the very moment that the ball left the player's hand (Fig. 5.9).[12]

---

[12] In a later study, Aglioti et al. worked again with the three groups composed by expert watchers, elite players and novices, showing them a set of video clips of the same duration as in the original experiment. This time, however, the videos

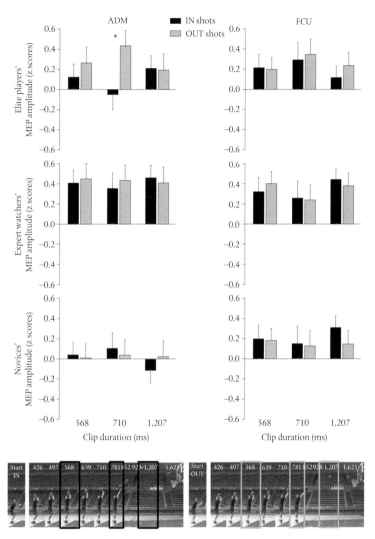

Fig. 5.9 Corticospinal activation during observation of basket shots that finish either IN or OUT of the hoop. The MEP were recorded from the *abductor digiti minimi* (ADM) and the *flexor carpi ulnaris* (FCU) at three clip durations, 568, 781, and 1,207 ms. Higher activation during the observation of OUT as compared with IN shots at the 781 ms clip was found only in the elite players (adapted from Aglioti et al., 2008).

Taken as a whole, these data show that visual expertise alone is not sufficient to guarantee a better performance in predicting the outcome of an action, especially when the critical information basically regards the motor components (the position of the hand, arm, body during the shot). On the other hand, motor expertise not only guarantees greater accuracy in predicting the outcome of an observed action, but also displays its predictive power right from the very early phases of the action.[13]

In all these studies, the role of motor expertise has been investigated by contrasting individuals with different skills, be they

showed two female volleyball players, filmed from in front and from the rear while executing volleyball floating services (Urgesi et al., 2012). Half of the clips started from the beginning of the action and lasted until the instant at which the player's hand touched the ball; the other half showed the initial trajectory of the ball from when it left the player's hand to when it was approximately at the height of the net. The outcome was that when the groups watched the videos showing only the initial phase of the action, the predictions of the elite players were more accurate than those of the novices, but also than those of the expert watchers (this was especially evident when they observed the action filmed from the rear). The expert watchers, on the other hand, when watching the video clips of the initial phase of the action, were never more accurate in their predictions than the novices. When the groups watched the videos showing the initial trajectory of the ball, the elite players were once again more accurate than the novices, but so were the expert watchers, especially when the trajectory was filmed from the rear.

[13] There is a vast literature regarding the contribution of motor expertise to the ability of athletes in various sports (from badminton to cricket, tennis to rugby, not to mention football) to predict the outcome of an action they are observing from the earliest phases. Among others, see Abernethy (2008) on badminton, Weissensteiner and collaborators (2008) on cricket, Farrow and Abernethy (2003) on tennis, Jackson and collaborators (2006) on rugby, Tomeo et al. (2013) on football. The fMRI study run by Martin Wright et al. (2010) is also worthy of mention; the authors demonstrate how expert badminton players recruit areas endowed with the mirror property when they are asked to predict the outcome of a serve, particularly when they have to rely on the initial phases of the action. Bishop and colleagues conducted a similar study on soccer (2013). For those interested in further reading on this topic, we recommend a study by Shiffrar and Heinen (2011), who have written at length on the role of motor expertise in the ability to understand when actions are feigned, an ability that is particularly useful for athletes (see also Shiffrar, 2011).

motor or visual. However, there is another fairly simple means of ascertaining if and to what extent motor expertise can influence our perceptual judgement of an observed action. We all have a motor expertise that is greater for our own actions than for those of others, whatever the kind of action. What happens, for example, when we have to identify an observed action goal or predict its outcome, if part of the actions that are presented are actions we ourselves have executed? Imagine for a moment that you are filmed while executing a certain task, and the resulting video has been cut so that only the initial phases of what you are doing are visible. You are shown this video, and videos of other people doing the same task, edited in the same way. If you were asked to predict the outcome of the observed actions based on watching the initial phases, would your predictions regarding the outcome of your own actions and those of others be equally accurate? Or would your prediction of the outcome of your own actions be more accurate, even if those outcomes should be no different from those resulting from the actions of others?

According to our hypothesis, the congruence between the visual representation of the observed action and the corresponding motor representation is greater when you yourself have executed the action as opposed to when it has been executed by someone else, even if that person has your same level of experience in that particular task, therefore it is to be expected that when the action you are observing is yours, the sensorimotor transformations characteristic of mirror responses will facilitate the identification of the action and the prediction of its outcome. More than one study has proved this to be the case.

One such study was conducted by Günther Knoblich and Rüdiger Flach; they asked a group of approximately one hundred participants to throw darts at a dartboard. They started with a motor training session; when the participants reached a certain level of ability, the authors filmed them and created three videos from the footage. In the first, the participants were completely visible while throwing the darts; in the second, their bodies were visible, but not their faces; in the third, only the arms throwing the darts were visible. None of the videos included the trajectory of the darts, only the act of throwing them. A few days later the participants were shown the videos: each person saw two videos, one showing their own performance, the other the performance of another person. They were organized into pairs, with one person seeing the video of their own performance first, while the other person saw the video of someone else's performance first. The task consisted in predicting whether the dart would land in the top, middle, or bottom of the target. The results showed that the participants were able to predict the outcome of the throw with a good level of accuracy from all three video sets; what was particularly interesting was that the level of accuracy was greater when they watched the footage of their own actions.[14]

---

[14] In a later study, Knoblich et al. asked a group of participants to copy a series of symbols by hand on a tablet, checking their accuracy with an image on a computer screen (Knoblich et al., 2002). A week later, the participants took an identification task involving various samples of writing. The task required the participant to look at the first stroke of a given symbol (for example, the number 2) and decide if it was free standing, or whether it would be accompanied by other strokes making up the symbol (the number 2). The participants were organized into pairs so that half of the samples given to each person were in their own writing and half in that of another person. The participants were not told that samples of their own writing were included in those they were given. The authors found that their participants were accurate in identifying strokes that made up a symbol and in predicting which strokes would follow only when they themselves had penned the strokes; when judging the strokes made by other participants they simply guessed. Fani Loula et al. at Rutgers University obtained similar results from a study using point-lights. They found that when their participants

What happens if mirror responses are interfered with?

What we have seen so far suggests that the sensorimotor trans-formations characteristic of mirror responses play a distinctive role in understanding action, making it possible to identify action goals and to realize that the action being observed is directed to one or more of them. However, our claim appears to be corrob-orated by yet another line of evidence based on rTMS (repetitive TMS) studies.

rTMS can be applied at high (>2 Hz) or low (0.2–1 Hz) frequency. When applied at low frequency (typically 1 Hz), it reduces cortical excitability, both at the application site and in the functionally cor-related areas for a duration similar to that of the actual stimulation. If, as we have claimed, the sensorimotor transformations charac-teristic of mirror responses play a distinctive role in understanding action, applying low-frequency rTMS to the motor cortical areas known to be endowed with the mirror property while observing actions should affect action goal identification.

Marcello Costantini and colleagues at the Universities of Chieti and of Milano carried out a rTMS experiment in order to test this prediction (Costantini, Ambrosini, Cardellicchio et al., 2014).

were asked to identify various kinds of actions represented by a number of point-light markers shown in a video, they were more accurate when the actions being observed were their own rather than those executed by people they knew (Loula et al., 2005). A later experiment conducted at Rutgers, this time by Prasad and Shiffrar (2009), excluded that such accuracy is to be attributed exclusively to visual sensitivity to self-generated action. The significant finding from this experiment was that the participants were more accurate in recognizing their own actions when the presentation was allocentric, regardless, more or less, of whether they were seen from a frontal or rear view. As we always see the actions we execute in the first person, it is unlikely that this effect can be attributed exclusively to visual familiarity with our own actions, but rather to the involvement of the motor processes and representations that are responsible for them.

It is common knowledge that when picking up an object, such as a mug for example, your gaze usually reaches it long before your hands do, due to rapid eye movements (saccades) which allow you to bring your desired mug onto the fovea (Hayhoe & Ballard, 2005; Land, 2009). The saccades proactively individuate the action target and extract the motorically relevant information such as position, orientation, size, and shape from it so that the grasping movements can be monitored and finally executed (Johansson et al., 2001). Most interestingly, a number of studies have shown that proactive saccades are present also when the grasping is being observed rather than executed. A particularly interesting experiment conducted by Randall Flanagan and Roland Johansson was published in *Nature* in 2003. The authors found that their participants showed a proactive eye-hand coordination both when building a construction with small wooden blocks themselves and when watching someone else doing the same (Flanagan & Johansson, 2003). According to the authors, while their participants were watching the grasping action, they were recruiting the same motor processes and representations they would have brought into play had they themselves been executing the action. When they were doing the building themselves, those processes and representations triggered proactive saccadic movements to identify possible goals. The same happened when they were watching the actions being carried out by others; their saccadic movements allowed them to individuate the action targets of the people they were watching.[15]

---

[15] After this seminal research by Flanagan and Johansson, a number of studies were conducted with the aim of systematically investigating the proactivity of saccadic movements while watching actions, such as grasping or moving an object, that normally require a considerable degree of eye-hand coordination.

Costantini and colleagues went a step further in this line of research. They applied low-frequency rTMS at 1 Hz for approximately fifteen minutes to three target areas located in the participants' left-brain hemisphere. These areas were the premotor ventral cortex (PMv), an area that, as we have mentioned before, is involved in the motor representation of grasping actions and possesses the mirror property; the posterior section of the superior temporal sulcus (pSTS), which contains a series of high-level visual areas encoding biological movements; the frontal eye field (FEF) that controls saccadic movements. Before and after the rTMS session the participants were asked to watch a video showing a hand reaching for and grasping one of two differently sized objects. The larger of the two required a whole hand prehension, the smaller a precision grip. In fifty percent of the videos, the preshaping of the hand was clearly visible during the hand lift-off, as normally happens. In the remaining fifty percent, there was no preshaping of the hand which however, closed into a fist, followed the same trajectory as before and only opened when it was positioned above the object. The participants were not given any particular instructions other than to watch the video carefully, nor did they know in advance which of the objects would be grasped. The recording of eye movements made before the rTMS session showed that the participants were much quicker and more accurate in identifying the target of the action being observed when watching the video with the preshaped hand rather than the one showing the closed fist (Fig. 5.10).

For further reading we recommend Rotman et al. (2006), Webb et al. (2010), and Ambrosini et al. (2011), among others.

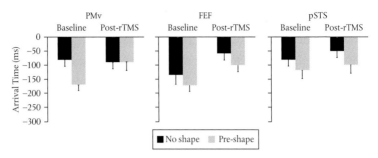

Fig. 5.10 Arrival time of gaze behaviour in the experimental conditions prior to and after the application of rTMS to the PMv, FEF, and pSTS. Only repeated stimulation of the PMv had a significant effect on the proactive gaze behaviour (adapted from Costantini, Ambrosini, Cardellicchio et al., 2014).

This changed after the rTMS session; repeated stimulation of the PMv resulted in a significant decrease of the proactivity of the saccadic movements when the participants were shown a hand that was preshaped from lift-off. Not only, this decrease in the proactivity was so marked that the participants took the same length of time to identify the target both when the hand was preshaped for grasping and when it was closed in a fist. This did not occur after stimulation of the FEF and pSTS; stimulation of these areas did have an effect but it was not specific, and did not selectively interfere with the ability to identify the type of prehension that the hand would assume and consequently which object would turn out to be the target (Fig. 5.10).

Taken together, these data suggest that the proactivity of the observer's eye movements depends primarily on the ability to use motor information regarding the preshaped grip, starting from the first phase of the task. The mirror response of the PMv and the corresponding sensorimotor transformation would therefore play a key role in the possibility of using this information, allowing identification of the goal of the observed action and its related target. If the ability to motorically represent the observed action is impaired even for just a few minutes, this will impact on the possibility of capturing the relevant motor information necessary to identify the observed action goal and predict its outcome.[16]

Cosimo Urgesi and colleagues at the University of Udine and of Rome's La Sapienza University obtained somewhat similar results from a rTMS study that investigated whether and to what extent the PMv played a distinctive role in identifying action goals (Urgesi, Candidi, Ionta et al., 2007). The participants were given a two-choice match-to-sample discrimination task showing actions that could be identified by the goals and bodily shaping. The stimulation was applied both to the PMv and the extrastriate body area (EBA), typically involved in the high-order processing of visual information relative to bodily movements and features (Downing et al., 2001; Peelen et al., 2006). The contrast between the two stimulations revealed a double dissociation; stimulation of the PMv diminished the participants' ability to accurately identify whether the actions were identical or had different goals but had no effect on their ability to identify the body parts involved. On the other hand, reduction of the EBA's excitability resulted in the participants being less accurate in their identification of the body

---

[16] The notion that the proactivity of the observer's gaze depends largely on their ability to motorically represent the action being observed has been corroborated by further studies that have showed how gaze proactivity can be significantly reduced by a number of purely motor factors, such as the inability to execute the action being observed while observing it (Ambrosini et al., 2012), the fact of perceiving that the target of the action being observed is out of the agent's reach (Costantini et al., 2012b) and finally, the fact of executing an action that is congruent or incongruent with the action being observed (Costantini et al., 2012a).

parts involved in the action without interfering with their ability to identify the corresponding goals.[17]

Subsequently, Ayse Pinar Saygin and colleagues at University College London used an rTMS protocol, known as continuous Theta Burst Stimulation (cTBS), which consists of short bursts of three TMS impulses of 50 Hz repeated at 200 ms, that usually results in a lessening of the cortical excitability of the area to which it is applied (van Kemenade et al., 2012). They stimulated the PMv and the posterior portion of the superior temporal sulcus (pSTS), which is involved in the visual representation of biological movements. Their participants were presented with brief video frames showing point-light displays for various activities (walking,

---

[17] Matteo Candidi et al. applied rTMS to the PMv and EBA in an identification task involving actions executed with biomechanically possible or impossible kinematics (Candidi et al., 2008). A comparison of the stimulations revealed that reducing the excitability of the PMv (but not of the EBA) negatively impacted the accuracy with which the participants judged the biomechanically possible actions; no impact was found on the biomechanically impossible actions. Another study conducted by Urgesi et al. at University College London (Urgesi, Calvo-Merino, Haggard et al., 2007) further corroborated the notion that PMv and EBA play different roles in representing bodily actions. It is well known that it is easier to identify a particular posture that could be involved in executing a certain action if the picture shows the body in a regular head up rather than head down position. There is a simple explanation for this: the perceptual identification of body posture is based on the processing of global configurations and not on specifically local aspects. The former, but not the latter, change as the orientation of the body changes. Urgesi et al. showed that applying rTMS to the PMv resulted in a deterioration of the ability to identify body postures only when they were presented in the normal position (i.e. head up), while repeated stimulation of the EBA caused a decreased ability to identify them when they were presented in the opposite mode (i.e. head down). This would suggest that PMv plays a key role in the processing of global configurations that facilitate the identification of body postures involved in action, while at the same time assisting with the identification of the goal with which the various postures appear to be connected. The EBA, on the other hand, appears to play an important role in the representation of more specifically local aspects of the various body parts, facilitating their identification in terms of identity.

running, kicking, taking a step forward or backward, side stepping) before and after stimulation. In fifty per cent of the frames, the point-light patterns were scrambled to conserve the same movements locally, which meant that the global configuration of the action was lost. The task consisted in recognizing whether an action had been executed. It was interesting to see how stimulation of the PMv resulted in a decrease in the accuracy of the participants' performance, as evidenced by an increase in the number of 'false alarms', in which the participants tended to erroneously identify actions even when the point-lights were scrambled and did not represent any action at all, in spite of conserving a semblance of movement. Stimulation of the pSTS however did not produce any effect. These findings indicate that visual representations, even of higher order, may be insufficient for the identification of observed actions. Indeed, they need to be integrated with the motor processes and representations evoked by mirror responses.

Finally, further evidence that the sensorimotor transformations characteristic of mirror responses play a distinctive role in identifying the goal of the action being observed came from a cTBS study conducted by John Michael of the University of Aarhus and the Wellcome Trust of London (Michael et al., 2014). They applied cTBS to their participants' left premotor cortex before having them complete a pantomime-recognition task in which half of the trials were based on pantomimed hand actions, and the other half on pantomimed mouth actions. The authors stimulated, in separate sessions, the sectors of the premotor cortex where the hand and the mouth (respectively more dorsal and more ventral in position) are represented. A comparison of the two sessions revealed a double dissociation: stimulation of the sector of the premotor cortex responsible for hand movement representation resulted in a decrease in the accuracy with which the participants identified observed actions executed with the hand; this effect was not present when the observed actions were executed with the mouth. In contrast, stimulation of the sector of the premotor cortex responsible for mouth movement representation affected participants' accuracy in identifying observed actions executed with the mouth; this effect was absent when the observed actions were executed with the hand.

What can we learn from lesions of areas with mirror properties?

The studies we have examined in the preceding section show how a temporary alteration of the excitability of the areas possessing the mirror property has a significant impact on the ability to understand an observed action. But what happens in brain-damaged patients, patients with lesions that directly involve areas endowed with the mirror property? If our claim that the sensorimotor transformations characteristic of mirror responses play a key role in understanding action is correct, then it is to be expected that these lesions might interfere not only with the ability to represent a given action motorically when executed personally, but also with the ability to understand it when it is executed by others. According to our claim, in fact, the latter ability may in many cases depend on the former.

Various studies seem to corroborate this. Daniel Tranel and colleagues at the University of Iowa ran a study with brain-damaged patients in which they found a clear association between the presence of lesions in the parieto-frontal areas of the left hemisphere, known to possess the mirror property, and difficulty in obtaining a normal score on tasks in which they had to use their sensori-motor abilities to identify the actions they were asked to observe or to compare (Tranel et al., 2003). In particular, there were patients who had great difficulty in understanding if one action was noisier than another, or which of two actions required a given movement or which of the two was more tiring; other patients struggled to indicate which of three actions was the least pertinent, others again performed below par on both tasks.

Similar results have been obtained by Peter Brugger and colleagues, working with two patients with congenital bilateral aplasia (Funk et al., 2005). One of the patients experienced vivid phantom movement sensations in both arms and hands, while the other did not. They asked the two patients and a group of control subjects to judge the direction of an apparent rotatory movement induced by seeing a rapid sequence of two images of a person extending their hand in two different positions. When the interval between the presentation of the two images was extremely short, both the patients and the control subjects tended to prefer the shortest path motions even if these implied a violation of biomechanical constraints. In contrast, when the interval between presentation of the images was sufficiently long, the two patients perceptually judged the apparent rotatory movement differently. Indeed, while the patient with no phantom limb movement sensation still reported perceiving the rotatory movement as being that of the shortest path even though it was anatomically impossible, the patient with phantom limb movement sensation perceived the rotatory movement in exactly the same way as the control subjects, i.e. as the longer path, which did not involve any violation of the biomechanical constraints. This finding was in line with previous studies demonstrating that the motor processes and representations evoked in the observer shape their perceptions only when the interval between the images was compatible with the execution of the action (Shiffrar & Freyd, 1990; Stevens et al., 2000). It is worth noting that motor processes and representations concerning missing limbs have been shown to be spared in aplasic patients with phantom limb movement sensations only (Mercier et al., 2006). This would explain why they might perceptually judge an observed action similarly to control subjects and differently from aplasic patients who have no phantom limb movement sensation. Their (spared) ability to represent that action impacted motorically on how they experienced the action when observing others executing it.

More recently, Mariella Pazzaglia and colleagues at Rome's La Sapienza University reported the case of apraxic patients with lesions in their left parieto-frontal areas (Pazzaglia, Smania, Corato et al., 2008). These patients not only had difficulty in executing or imitating manual tasks involving the use of instruments such as a hammer and nail, or in executing symbolic communication gestures such as shaping the hand to form the signal for hitching a ride, they also had difficulty when observing manual actions using instruments or symbolic gestures and then judging whether they were executed correctly. The authors ran another study, comparing the performance on action execution and action understanding in apraxic patients with left hemisphere brain damage in their parieto-frontal regions (Pazzaglia, Pizzamiglio, Pes et al., 2008). Their participants showed various deficits in executing actions: some had difficulty only in executing manual tasks, others only with tasks executed by mouth, others again had problems with both. The comprehension task consisted in listening to sounds linked to an action executed with the hands (e.g. clapping) or with the mouth (e.g. whistling) and then identifying them from four images. It was interesting to see that the participants who had difficulty in executing manual actions were also less accurate in identifying the actions linked to the sounds produced by such actions, and an analogous situation was found in the patients who had difficulty in executing actions by mouth (Fig. 5.11).

Valentina Moro and colleagues at the University of Verona and Rome's La Sapienza University obtained similar results from a study based on the paradigm used by Urgesi and colleagues

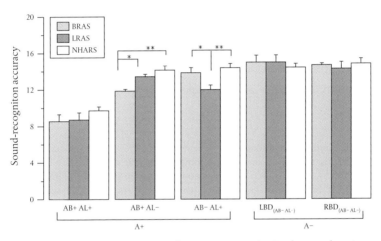

Fig. 5.11 Accuracy in action-sound recognition in brain-damaged patients with (A+) and without (A–) apraxia. The stimuli consisted in sounds produced by buccofacial actions (BRAS), sounds produced by hand-arm actions (LRAS), and sounds resulting from non-human events (NHARS). The apraxic patients were grouped into those who were apraxic for actions requiring use of the upper limbs but not of the mouth (AB– AL+), those whose apraxia affected actions executed by the mouth but not by the upper limbs (AB + AL–), and those who showed both types of apraxia (AB + AL+). The apraxic patients turned out to be less accurate only in recognizing actions associated with their own type of apraxia. No deficit was found in brain-damaged patients without apraxia (adapted from Pazzaglia, Pizzamiglio, Pes et al., 2008).

(Urgesi, Candini, Ionta et al., 2007). They recruited a group of brain-damaged patients with lesions principally in their frontal or temporo-occipital regions to participate in tasks consisting of identifying an action or the body parts involved in that action, after which they compared the accuracy of the responses (Moro et al., 2008). The patients with the frontal lesions had difficulty in identifying the observed actions but were able to identify the body parts involved, whereas the patients with posterior lesions had difficulty in identifying the body parts, but were able to identify the actions. To be more specific, the difficulties in identifying the observed actions were strongly associated with lesions of the premotor ventral cortex, while those in identifying the body parts were associated with lesions of the occipital and middle-temporal gyrus, situated in a region corresponding to the EBA, which is known to be involved in the higher order visual representation of various body parts.[18]

---

[18] The finding that lesions of the parieto-frontal regions can be associated with deficits in action production and comprehension is supported also by a study conducted by Andrea Serino and colleagues at the University of Bologna. The aim of their experiment was to compare the degree of accuracy in action comprehension tasks achieved by brain-damaged patients (Serino et al., 2009). Some of these patients were hemiplegic with lesions of the parieto-frontal regions; others were hemiplegic with temporo-parietal lesions. The brain-damaged patients and a control group of healthy volunteers were shown brief videos with a limited number of point-lights representing a series of transitive manual actions (grasping a bottle, turning a key, using a hammer) or symbolic-communicative gestures (waving goodbye with the hand, shaking the index finger from left to right to indicate negation, tapping the forehead with a finger to express frustration, 'How stupid!'). The video clips were manipulated so the actions could be shown either as they had occurred or as a specular image, as if they had been produced by the other hand. It was interesting to see that the brain-damaged patients were in general less accurate than the control group in identifying actions, but it was even more interesting to see that the hemiplegic patients were significantly less accurate in their judgement when the actions were presented as a specular image, giving the impression that they were being produced by the arm and hand that these patients were unable to use due to their hemiplegia.

Emotions

In the preceding section, we focused on the various lines of evidence corroborating our claim that mirror responses play a key role in understanding the actions that we see other people executing. Indeed, on the whole the data we have reviewed above indicates that how we identify the goal(s) of an observed action often depends on how we represent that goal (or those goals) motorically. It follows that, if for some reason (such as another action being carried out at the same time, the acquisition of new expertise, the presence of transitory or permanent lesions) we change this way of representing that action goal (or those action goals), our way of understanding and judging the observed action will also change.

We have been talking here about the action domain, but we know there is evidence that mirror responses also exist in the domains of emotion and vitality forms. In particular, in Chapter 3 we have seen that the anterior portion of the insula (AI), the amygdale and the pregenual anterior cingulate cortex (pACC) possess the mirror property, respectively processing our own reactions of disgust, fear, and laughter and those of others. When we observe other people expressing these emotions, we recruit the same visceromotor processes and representations we would have brought into play had we been experiencing them ourselves. Assuming this to be correct, it is to be expected that, as with actions which have no emotional significance, visceromotor transformations characteristic of mirror responses will also play a distinctive role in understanding the emotions of others, allowing us to identify other people's expressions and recognize the kind of emotion they are experiencing. In the following pages we will show that there is indeed evidence, most of which deriving from clinical studies of cerebral lesions, to support our claim at least as far as expressions of disgust and fear are concerned.

The case of the missing sense of disgust

In Chapter 3 we saw how fMRI experiments, stimulation studies and intracranial registration show that the ventral portion of AI possesses the mirror property for the processes and representations involved in disgust (pp. 95–101). We suggested that AI's mirror responses would determine a transformation of visual representations of disgusted expressions seen on other people's faces into the processes and representations that are responsible for visceral and motor reactions that contribute to shaping our own experience of disgust. Due to this transformation, visual information processed in the temporal lobe reaches the cortical and subcortical centres generally activated by the natural stimuli that evoke reactions of disgust. When we see a grimace of disgust, it triggers a process recruiting visceromotor representations similar to those that would have been recruited if we ourselves had been experiencing it.

In the following pages, we will explore the claim that this recruitment plays a distinctive role in understanding other people's disgust, allowing us to identify their reaction and realize that it is indeed a reaction of disgust. If this claim is correct, lesions of the AI would interfere not only with our ability to represent an emotion such as disgust visceromotorically and experience it personally, but it would also impair our ability to understand disgust for what it is when we see it in the facial expression of another person.

Evidence of this emerged from a study conducted by Andrew Calder and colleagues at the University of Cambridge and published on *Nature Neuroscience* over twenty years ago (Calder et al., 2000). Their patient N.K. had suffered a left hemisphere lesion that had badly damaged the AI and the putamen; his scores on various tests to evaluate his ability to recognize emotions were in the norm for anger, fear, sadness, happiness, surprise, but revealed that he had difficulty with disgust. The same results emerged for non-verbal acoustic stimuli or prosodies with specific emotional content; the patient continued to have difficulty when asked to recognize those linked to disgust, such as the sound of retching. It is important to note that these difficulties could not be attributed to a semantic deficit. In fact, the patient had no problem identifying scenes representing situations that are typically associated with a given emotion, such as disgust at a filthy toilet, so it was evident that he had a good command of the concepts linked to the various emotions, including disgust. On the other hand, and what is most interesting for our purposes, when faced with stimuli that could plausibly evoke disgust, his reactions were significantly different compared to the norm. His performance on questionnaires designed to measure experience intensity was notably inferior to that of the control group, particularly when the questions regarded food, animals, excrements, and exposed innards, but his scores on fear and anger were aligned with those of the control group. The patient's difficulty in identifying and understanding other people's expressions of disgust was therefore associated with a lack of his personal experience of this emotion, which, in the words of the authors themselves, would indicate that 'the neural substrates of emotional experience are engaged during recognition of emotion expressed by others' (Calder et al., 2000, p. 1078).

Ralph Adolphs and colleagues at Iowa University reported a similar case (Adolphs et al., 2003). Their patient, B., had suffered a vast bilateral lesion involving the cortical regions, including the AI. In spite of the fact that he had no deficit in visual perception of faces, he had serious difficulty in recognizing expressions of disgust when shown to him as static images (photographs), or as dynamic facial expressions produced by the experimenter. Indeed, when faced with an experimenter producing various emotional reactions as naturally as possible, B. was able to identify them all, with the sole exception of disgust. The authors also did an extra test to see if B. was able to recognize expressions of disgust on the faces of other people, executing actions that are normally associated with a strong sense of disgust. They took a bite of food and then spat it out with a grimace of disgust, accompanied by the sound of retching. B's reactions were really surprising and showed just how little he understood of what the experimenters trying to convey. He was totally indifferent and even, in one case, remarked that the food the experimenter had tasted was 'delicious'. In this case also, the most interesting finding was that B. seemed to be incapable of experiencing disgust himself. He was able to eat all kinds of substances, even the most inedible, and showed no sign of disgust when shown pictures of food writhing with worms or beetles that usually provoke a strong reaction.

The notion that the ability to recognize other people's expressions of disgust may relate to the ability to visceromotorically represent one's own disgust and experience it personally, seems to be supported by a study conducted by Andreas Hennenlotter and colleagues at the University of München on a number of subjects genetically at risk of developing Huntington's chorea, a hereditary neurogenerative disease caused by the mutation of the HTT

(IT15) gene (Hennenlotter et al., 2005). Earlier studies had shown that patients with symptoms of Huntington's disease had difficulty in identifying facial expressions linked to disgust (see, for example, Sprengelmeyer et al., 1996), and similar difficulties had been found in people with a mutation of IT15 but who still did not show symptoms of the disease (Gray et al., 1997). Hennelotter and colleagues designed an experiment to investigate the neural substrate involved in these difficulties, exploring the cortical activations and the behavioural performance of nine presymptomatic carriers of the mutant IT15 gene in recognizing facial expressions of disgust in other people, and of nine healthy subjects as a control group. They found that the activation of the AI in the group with the mutant gene while observing grimaces of disgust on the faces of others was significantly weaker compared to that of the control group. Moreover, while a much stronger activation in this area emerged in the control group when observing expressions of disgust compared to a neutral expression, it was completely absent in the presymptomatic group. It was interesting to see that the data obtained at a cerebral level correlated with the performance of identification of emotional expressions at the behavioural level: the presymptomatic group were notably less accurate than the control subjects when identifying grimaces of disgust on the faces of other people. This was not the case for other emotional expressions (e.g. happiness, sadness, joy, and fear), where there was no difference in accuracy between the two groups.

Christopher Kipps and colleagues at the University of Cambridge obtained similar results from a voxel-based morphometry study that they designed to assess whether differences in grey matter volume were related to impairments in the identification of other people's emotional expressions in presymptomatic carriers of the mutant IT15 gene (Kipps et al., 2007). The results did in fact show a significant correlation between the volume of grey matter in the AI and the performance on tasks involving the identification of grimaces of disgust by these subjects. Once again, there was no similar correlation with other emotional expressions, nor was it present in the control group.[19]

More recently, Costanza Papagno and colleagues at the University of Milano-Bicocca in collaboration with the Unit of Surgical Neuro-Oncology of the Humanitas Research Hospital led by Lorenzo Bello, studied the role of the AI in identifying facial expressions of disgust during awake surgery (Papagno et al., 2016). It is common clinical practice to keep the patient awake during resection of brain tumours in order to assess the functional role of the cerebral regions around the tumour that may be involved in the surgery. One way of doing this, which produces functional maps with an excellent spatiotemporal resolution, is to use direct electric stimulation to inactivate the regions closest to the tumour. In their study, Papagno and colleagues directly stimulated the insula in a group of patients while they were doing a classic emotion expression identification task. The patients were unaware of the stimulation, which was done while they were being shown images of faces with various expressions. The authors discovered that stimulating the insula significantly interfered with the patients' performance on identifying expressions of disgust, but with none of the other expressions. During stimulation, the patients were less accurate in judging the expressions of disgust they saw, but their performance

---

[19] A similar correlation between deficits in understanding other people's disgust and a reduction of the grey matter of the ventral portion of the AI was also found by Joshua Woolley et al. in a study on patients affected by frontotemporal dementia (Woolley et al., 2015).

on identifying other emotional expressions was not affected. This finding acquires even greater significance considering that disgust is one of the easiest expressions to recognize; in fact, it is normally identified correctly in 93.10% of cases (Broks et al., 1998; Young et al., 2002).

While further research is necessary, the studies we have reviewed above provide good reason to believe that the sensori-visceromotor transformations induced by the mirror responses of the AI play a distinctive role in understanding other peoples' disgust, allowing us to identify the observed emotional expression and recognize that it is expressive of disgust. The nature and function of this understanding will be discussed in the next chapter; for the time being, we will just say that evidence in favour of our claim that mirror responses contribute to understanding other people is not sourced exclusively from the action domain. It also comes from the emotion domain.

Feeling no fear, but knowing what it is

The claim that the visceromotor transformations characteristic of mirror responses play a distinctive role in understanding other people's emotions is also supported by studies conducted on reactions of fear. In Chapter 3 we saw that the amygdala possesses the mirror property for this emotional reaction (pp. 102–106). Its mirror responses would involve a transformation of the visual and acoustic representations concerning fear expressed by others into the processes and representations that trigger the physiological and motor responses that are normally induced by the processing of threatening and dangerous stimuli and contribute to shaping our own experience of fear. Our claim is that this sensori-visceromotor transformation would enable us to understand other people's expressions of fear.

As in the case for disgust, the data in support of our claim come mainly from studies on patients with focal lesions. Adolphs and colleagues studied a patient, S.M., for many years. This patient had developed Urbach–Wiethe disease at the age of 10, with calcification of the amygdala in both hemispheres (see, among others, Adolphs et al., 1994; Adolphs et al., 1995; Adolphs et al., 1999; Feinstein et al., 2011).[20] Her social behaviour showed an affective imbalance, she had evident difficulty in identifying potentially dangerous situations and acting accordingly. Antonio Damasio discussed this case extensively in his *The Feeling of What Happens: Body and Emotion in the Making of Consciousness;* he observed that:

> S.M. does not experience fear in the same way you and I would in a situation that would normally induce it. At a purely intellectual level she *knows* what fear is supposed to be, what should cause it, and even what to do in situations of fear, but little or none of that intellectual baggage, so to speak, is of any use to her in the real world. (Damasio, 1999, p. 66. our italics)

Stimuli that normally induce fear, such as the sudden appearance of a snake or a spider, caused her surprise at most, but she never actually felt fear, nor did such stimuli cause her to adopt the

---

[20] As is well known, it is unusual to find patients with bilateral lesions of the amygdala. S.M.'s case was of particular interest because, unlike other patients, her bilateral lesions were mostly confined to this region. We would recommend the excellent chapter by Feinstein et al. (2016) in *Living without an Amygdala,* edited by David Amaral and Ralph Adolphs (Amaral & Adolphs, 2016) for readers who are interested in S.M.'s case, which is probably the best documented neuropsychological case study of all time.

usual caution or avoidance tactics. This was true even when she was exposed to situations or places known to evoke fear or terror, as when she was taken to visit Waverly Hills Sanatorium, which came to fame in the television series *Ghost Busters* and is still considered to be one of the ghostliest hospital premises in the United States. For S.M.'s visit to the sanatorium, the researchers arranged for a realistic haunted house to be prepared, complete with elaborate decorations, spooky noises, and ghostly and ghastly monsters. When she was taken into the house, S.M. was thrilled when she heard unnerving noises or met strange beings, but showed no signs of nervousness or of alert. She was given a handheld electronic 'emotion diary' on which to record the level of her emotions daily for about three months, using around fifty terms associated with emotions. The only terms to which she attributed a minimum score were those directly or indirectly associated with fear, while the term to which she assigned the maximum score was 'fearless' (Feinstein et al., 2011).

This was also reflected in visceral and physiological reactions to potentially dangerous stimuli. In an emotional conditioning experiment in which S.M. took part, unlike the control subjects, she had no autonomic response at all (e.g. an increase in skin conductance) when presented with a conditioned stimuli with a negative emotive valence. On the contrary, there was no difference between her ability to learn and that of the control subjects; she had no difficulty in identifying the stimuli and providing accurate information regarding them (Bechara et al., 1995).

What we found particularly interesting was that there was a clear connection between S.M.'s inability to feel fear as most people do and her inability to correctly recognize fear in the facial expressions of others (Adolphs et al., 1995). When asked to evaluate the intensity of a fearful expression, she invariably tended to give a much lower score than that given by the control subjects, even when there was absolutely no doubt as to the significance of the facial expression in question.[21] In the cases in which she did give these expressions a high score, she classified them as surprise or anger, but not as fear.[22] She did not, however, have any problems with other emotional expressions nor did she exhibit impairment in identifying faces and features. When asked to elaborate on the expressions of fear she had not been able to identify as such, S.M. said she knew that they were emotional expressions but was not sure which emotion it was. Most of the time she opted for surprise or anger; in only one case did she say that she thought it might be fear. Finally, although she was a talented artist, S.M. appeared unable to depict expressions of fear, in spite of being perfectly capable of sketching faces with other emotional expressions. Nor was she able to imitate a grimace of fear. Damasio noted that her attempts [to imitate a grimace of fear] did not change her expression to any great degree and finally she had to admit that she just wasn't capable of producing an expression of fear. On the contrary, she had no difficulty in imitating an expression of surprise (Damasio,

---

[21] It is worthy of note that S.M.'s scores were significantly lower even than those of patients with unilateral lesions of the amygdala; in fact, there was no difference between the performance of these patients and that of the controls (Adolphs et al., 1995).

[22] The inability to recognize expressions of fear on the faces of other people can be problematical when living in a social environment. Adolphs et al. showed that patients with bilateral lesions of the amygdala, including S.M., tend to trust strangers, particularly if they have an unsavoury appearance, much more than healthy subjects do (Adolphs et al., 1999). It also emerged that S.M. did not have a normal perception of peripersonal space and showed no discomfort if a stranger stood too close to her, even if they came right up to her at nose-to-nose distance (Kennedy et al., 2009).

1999, p. 87), even though expressions of surprise are not so very different from expressions of fear.[23]

Sprengelmeyer and his colleagues described a similar case; their patient N.M., a fifty-year-old male, had been admitted to the Hospital of Bochum on return from an intercontinental trip, suffering from bilateral gliosis of the amygdala and a left thalamic

---

[23] Successively, S.M. took part in a study with a pair of monozygotic twins (A.M. and B.G.) suffering from bilateral focal lesions of the amygdala, to explore responses to interoceptive stimuli. Feinstein and colleagues discovered that inhaling a substance composed of 35% CO_2-evoked responses more or less connected with fear in all three subjects, albeit in different degrees. In fact, inhaling this substance caused panic attacks, dyspnoea, adverse behaviour (attempts to tear off the mask), and modifications of the patients' physiological state including changes in heartbeat and skin conductance. Sahib Khalsa and colleagues obtained similar results in another study with these twins, during which they received intravenous infusions of isoproterenol, an adrenergic beta stimulant similar to adrenaline that acts rapidly peripherally and is known to be a strong panicogen (Khalsa et al., 2016). Both twins showed signs of anxiety after the injection and B.G. suffered a panic attack. Two observations are in order here. Firstly, as the authors of both studies have pointed out, these results are an integration rather than a confutation of the data reported in the text, as the panic and anxiety experienced by the patients depended on the use of interoceptive stimuli, the processes of which take place along pathways that are at least partially independent of the functioning of the amygdala; this is not the case for the exteroceptive stimuli used in the studies we have reported here (see Feinstein et al., 2016 on this point). Secondly, even when the interoceptive stimuli were used, the fear and anxiety experienced by the patients was anomalous. In particular, it is important to note that S.M. reported that her experience while inhaling the CO_2 was completely new to her. The levels of anxiety and panic induced by inhaling this substance were higher than those experienced by the control group, and there was a greater increase in their heart rate and skin conductance; in addition, these effects occurred in the patients with brain lesions only after inhaling the CO_2, while the control group experienced them gradually, starting from when they saw the experimenters preparing the equipment. These findings seem to be in line with our claim that impairments of the visceromotor representations and first-hand experience of a given emotion can be associated with impairments in the understanding of that particular emotion when seen on the face of another person. They lead us to surmise that the possibility of mirror responses to reactions induced by interoceptive stimuli should be investigated, extending the range and reach of the visceromotor transformations characteristic of mirror responses to the observation of other people's facial expressions of fear.

lesion among other things. His scoring on questionnaires to evaluate situations and experiences that could cause fear on a range from one to five was significantly lower than the control group. N.M. himself admitted that he had rarely experienced fear; he delighted in remembering adventurous hunting expeditions along the Orinoco river and in Siberia, but when asked what he had felt when finding himself face to face with a jaguar or a stag he replied, 'excitement, never fear', and this was always the case when he found himself in potentially dangerous situations.

Like S.M., N.M. showed a clear association between a deficit in experiencing fear personally and an equally severe impairment in understanding expressions of fear on other people's faces. On a battery of tests to measure his ability to recognize facial expressions, body posture, and vocal expressions commonly associated with various emotions, he invariably scored significantly lower in identifying expressions of fear than on expressions related to other emotions.

Similar results were obtained in a collaborative study comparing different case studies involving a relatively large number of patients with bilateral damage to the amygdala; the objective was to ascertain whether bilateral amygdala damage impairs recognition of emotions, particularly fear, in facial expressions (Adolphs et al., 1999). The comparison showed that, overall, these patients had more difficulty in recognizing the expression of fear, and the difficulty was not so much in recognizing the facial expression as such but in recognizing it as expressing fear.[24]

---

[24] Other studies along similar lines include those conducted by Becker et al. (2011) and Bach et al. (2015). In the study run by Adolphs et al. (1999) there were differences, some of which quite marked, in the individual responses of the patients they tested, that can be only partially attributed to the site of the lesion.

Vitality Forms

The data we have seen so far corroborates our claim regarding the distinctive role that the sensorimotor and visceromotor transformations characteristic of mirror responses play respectively in the domains of action and emotion (specifically, in our case, of disgust and fear). However, in Chapter 4 we saw that there is evidence of the existence of mirror responses for vitality forms, the term we have borrowed from Daniel Stern. A number of recent studies have indeed shown that the posterior central part of the insula (DCI) appears to be involved in the affective modulation of actions, whether these are executed in the first person or are observed while being executed by other people (see pp. 130–138); as we have mentioned earlier, this modulation is more concerned with the form that characterizes the goal of the action rather than with the goal itself. When we observe other people executing an action, the sensory representations evoked by the sight of this action being executed with one particular vitality form rather than

Although this is not surprising given the differences in the patients' clinical histories and personalities, various explanations have been proposed. The authors themselves suggested that, although the amygdala plays a distinctive role in processing other people's facial expressions of fear, this does not exclude that this task could be executed with a certain degree of success using different strategies and resources, and following anatomical structures and routes as an alternative to the amygdala (Adolphs et al., 1999, p. 116). As we will see in the next chapter, these differences are in no way incompatible with our claim that the mirror responses of the amygdala play a key role in understanding other people's facial expressions of fear. , At least in some cases, this is not only because a practically normal understanding of other people's fearful expressions went hand in hand with an equally normal ability to visceromotorically represent fearful reactions and experience them personally (see, for example, the differences in the patients studied by Becker and collaborators, 2011 but also those studied by Khalsa and colleagues, 2016).

another are transformed into motor representations that imbue that action with that specific vitality form when we execute it ourselves. Our claim here is that if, when observing an action executed with a given vitality form, we recruit motor processes and representations similar to those we would have recruited had we been executing that action with that vitality form ourselves, then that recruitment may allow us to identify that vitality form as revelatory of the affective quality of the observed action.

In Chapter 4 we cited an fMRI study conducted by Di Cesare and colleagues at the University of Parma (Di Cesare et al., 2014). This study provided the first data in support of this claim. The participants were asked to watch pairs of very short video clips transmitted consecutively, showing two actors executing a series of actions with either the same or different action goals and vitality forms. Two tasks were set, the *What* task and the *How* task: in the first, the *What* task, the participants were asked to decide whether the action they were observing was the same or different (e.g. passing a bottle or giving a high five) without taking into consideration the vitality form involved, i.e. whether the action was executed gently or rudely. In the second, the *How* task, they were asked to decide whether the vitality form used was the same or different without taking into consideration which of the two actions was involved.

As was to be expected, in both tasks the analysis of the BOLD signal highlighted the activation of the frontoparietal areas that typically possess mirror properties for action goals. The interesting point here was that the contrast between the activations registered in the two tasks evidenced a significant activation of the DCI when the participants were asked to identify the vitality form of the observed action, regardless of the action goal (Fig. 5.12).

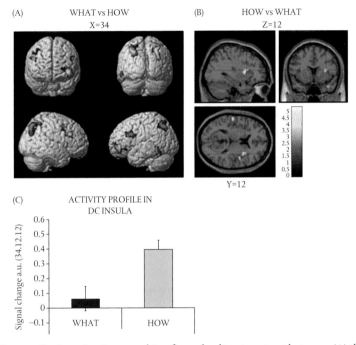

Fig. 5.12 Brain activations resulting from the direct contrast between (A) the *What* versus the *How* task and (B) the *How* versus the *What* task. (C) Activation profiles within the right DCI in the direct contrast between the *How* task versus the What task (adapted from Di Cesare et al., 2014).

The authors ran another study two years later in which the participants were asked to identify the vitality forms connected to certain actions they were asked to observe, such as passing a can of Coca-Cola, or the physical properties, such as speed, that characterized the execution of the action (Di Cesare, Valente, Di Dio et al., 2016). From a behavioural point of view, their study showed that when the participants were asked to identify either the vitality form characterizing the action (*very rude, rude, neutral, gentle, very gentle*) or the speed of its execution (*very fast, fast, average, slow, very slow*), they judged differently stimuli which actually were identical.

It was extremely interesting to see that this happened also at cerebral level; in fact, the comparison between the activation patterns of the insular cortex in response to the various vitality forms and those induced by the assessment of the speed indicated the presence (particularly in the right hemisphere) of voxels discriminating vitality forms compared to speed in the DCI (Fig. 5.13).

This suggests that the sensorimotor transformations triggered by the mirror responses of the dorso-central portion of the insula are involved in identifying the vitality form that characterizes how the observed action has been executed. Furthermore, and this is the point that interests us the most, studies conducted with participants diagnosed with autism spectrum disorder (ASD) show that identifying the vitality form that characterizes an action is, both at the cerebral and the cognitive level, different to and mostly independent of identifying the goal of the action, to the extent that one can exist without the other.

Magali Rochat and colleagues compared the performances of individuals diagnosed with ASD with those of control subjects matched for chronological and verbal age on recognition tasks regarding action goals and action vitality forms, similar to those used in the fMRI studies we have described earlier (Rochat et al., 2013). In the first task, they asked their participants to judge if the goals of two actions seen in rapid succession were the same or different; in the second, the participants had to decide whether the vitality forms of the two actions were identical or not. The two actions, in fact, could differ for either the action goal or the vitality form, or both the action goal and the vitality form could be different or they could be identical. On the first task, the performance of the subjects with ASD was not significantly less accurate than that of the controls, i.e. when the task required them to identify the

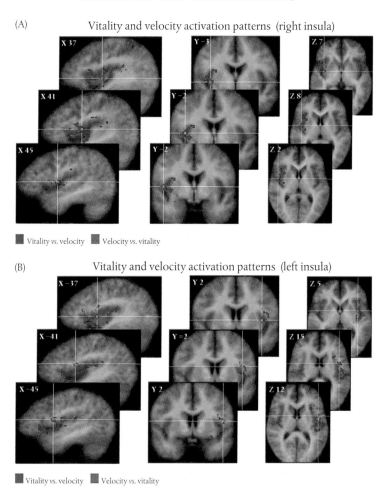

Fig. 5.13 Maps showing the most discriminative voxels for the perceptual difference of vitality forms (red) and speed (blue), in the right (A) and in the left (B) insula (adapted from Di Cesare, Valente, Di Dio et al., 2016).

goal of the actions and decide whether it was the same or different. However, when they were required to identify the vitality forms on the second task, the situation changed radically. As can be seen in Fig. 5.14 the subjects with ASD were much less accurate than

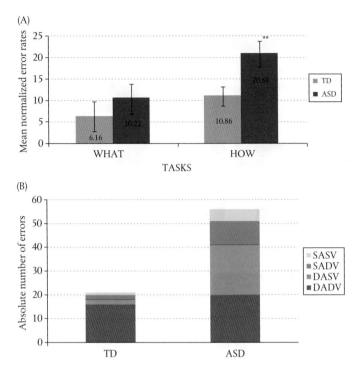

Fig. 5.14 The graph above (A) shows mean frequency of the errors made by ASD and control subjects (TD) on the goal (WHAT) or vitality form (HOW) identification task. The graph below (B) shows the distribution of errors in the HOW task among the four stimuli combinations for ASD and controls. SASV = same action, same vitality form; SADV = same action, different vitality form; DASV = different action, different vitality form; DADV = different action, different vitality form (adapted from Rochat et al., 2013).

the controls (A), in particular when they were required to identify the same vitality form in actions with different goals or to recognize that actions with similar goals exhibited a different vitality form (B).

This finding that the performance of subjects diagnosed with ASD does not differ from that of control subjects on the action goal identification task is extremely interesting and is in line with the results of a study conducted by Sonia Boria and colleagues. In this study, children diagnosed with ASD and a group of control subjects were asked to look at pictures with various hand-object interactions (such as a hand touching or grasping a pen or a glass) and then judge what the hand was doing and why it was doing it (if the hand grasped the object, was it going to use it for drinking from, or to move it?) (Boria et al., 2009). The ASD children did not have excessive difficulty in identifying the immediate goal of the action, whereas they found it more difficult to understand its distal goal, tending to let themselves be guided by the target object rather than by the observed action. For example, when the task involved a glass they had no difficulty in deciding whether the hand was going to grasp it or simply touch it, but when asked why the hand was grasping the glass, the answer was very often, 'to drink from it' even when the configuration of the grasp, with an approach from above, made this very unlikely.[25] Similar results were obtained

---

[25] This finding becomes even more significant when seen in the light of a study run by Luigi Cattaneo et al. The participants in their study, a group of children diagnosed with ASD and a control group of typically developing children (TD), were asked to execute actions such as lifting food to put it in their mouths or into a container, and then to watch other people executing the same actions. The activation of the mouth-opening mylohyoid muscle was recorded in both tasks (Cattaneo et al., 2007). The results showed that the typically developing children started activating this muscle during the reaching phase, when they picked up the food to carry it to their mouth. The muscle was not activated when they picked the food up to transfer it to a container, even when the container was fixed to their shoulder, not far from the mouth. A similar activation pattern was recorded when the children watched other people picking up a piece of food to lift it to their mouths or to put it in a container. In this case too, there was a significant activation of the mylohyoid muscle in the TD group when picking up the food to lift it to the mouth, but not when it was to be put in the container. The interesting point is that the results of the ASD group differed from those of the TD group on both tasks. They showed no activation of the mylohyoid muscle while reaching for the food, even when the task required it to be lifted to the mouth. The activation only occurred when the hand started on its trajectory to the mouth.

by Antonia Hamilton and colleagues. They showed that ASD children had no difficulty in imitating the goal of the action they were asked to watch, in fact they were able to do so even when the person performing the action did not achieve the intended goal (Hamilton et al., 2007).

As far as Rochat et al.'s second point is concerned, there are a number of studies which corroborate the view that individuals with ASD have difficulties in vitality form recognition. For example, Peter Hobson and Anthony Lee have shown that while the children with ASD who participated in their study were able to imitate the goal of the actions they observed quite adequately, they tended not to replicate the vitality forms that characterized them, particularly when they were not directly connected with the goal. The children were asked to imitate the following actions: tapping a pipe rack positioned on their shoulder with a wand, as if they were playing a violin; wiping their forehead with a piece of cloth; pressing a rubber stamp on a surface after inking it; using two fingers to press the head of a toy policeman to make it walk. The children with ASD were able to execute these actions just as well as the control group; however, if the actions were executed with

---

This indicates that the ASD children were not able to represent the action of reaching for and grasping an object motorically as part of a complex action with the goal of grasping the object to lift it to the mouth rather than to place it in a container. Therefore, it is not surprising that they did not activate the mylohyoid muscle when watching other people's grasping actions with the goal of lifting an object to the mouth rather than putting it in a container. As they do not have the ability to represent their own actions motorically, they were not able to recruit such representations when watching other people executing those same actions. This also explains why the participants in Boria et al.'s experiment had difficulty in identifying distal goals of an observed action, especially when the goal was not suggested by the target object itself.

a particular vitality form, say gently or rudely, most of the ASD group simply imitated the action but not the vitality form while the control group imitated both.

Some years later, Peter and Jessica Hobson obtained similar results from a study they designed to systematically investigate the ability of ASD children to imitate the vitality forms characterizing actions they were asked to observe (Hobson & Hobson, 2008). The authors used a set of relatively simple actions, testing the ability to imitate goal-directed actions on the one hand, and on the other the ability to imitate the vitality form used in executing the actions. They also distinguished between vitality forms that were not incidental to achieving the goal, vitality forms that were and vitality forms that constituted the goal or at least part of it. As in the previous study, the performance of the ASD children on the goal-directed imitation tasks did not differ from that of the control subjects; however, when required to imitate the vitality form of a given action, they did not perform as well as the control group, particularly when the vitality form was incidental to the goal of the action.

In a very recent study, Luca Casartelli and colleagues recorded the kinematics of ASD and TD children while they were performing placing and throwing actions with two different vitality forms (i.e. gentle and rude) (Casartelli, Cesareo, Biffi et al., 2020). The results showed that although ASD children were able to understand the concepts of rudeness and gentleness, and did try to follow the instructions to implement the corresponding vitality forms, they did not appear to express them motorically in the same way that the TD children did. Indeed, while TD children systematically varied their movement time to differentiate gentle from rude actions, with the latter being basically shorter in time than the former, ASD children tended to take approximately the same time when executing gentle and rude actions, with rude actions being even longer than gentle actions in around 30% of cases.

Interestingly, in a subsequent study, Casartelli and colleagues explored whether neurotypical adults may have difficulty in understanding vitality forms expressed by ASD children (Casartelli, Federici, Fumagalli, et al., 2020). Participants were presented with two videos showing two different types of actions (placing versus throwing) performed with two different vitality forms (rude versus gentle). Unknown to the participants, half the actions were executed by ASD children and the other half by TD children. The authors created the videos by extracting kinematic signals from their previous study. The participants were instructed to pay attention to how the action was executed (gently or rudely) and to judge the vitality form of the observed action, regardless of its goal, as quickly and accurately as possible. In the control condition, they had to pay attention to which action was executed (placing or throwing) and to judge the goal of the observed action, regardless of its vitality form, as quickly and accurately as possible. The results showed that the participants were much slower and less accurate in recognizing vitality forms when expressed by ASD children than when expressed by TD children. The effect was much more reduced in recognizing goals when the actions were executed by ASD children.

According to our claim, observing someone else acting with a given vitality form would involve a transformation of the sensory information concerning the observed action into processes and representations which would occur if the observers were expressing that vitality form themselves. If the observed actions match the internal representation of corresponding vitality forms, this would allow the observers to recognize them, as well as to track any related moods or affective states. The finding that ASD children represent vitality forms differently from TD children could explain why they have been shown to be impaired in recognizing and imitating vitality forms expressed by neurotypical individuals. But it also could explain why neurotypical adults turn out to have significant difficulty in understanding vitality forms expressed by ASD children. When observing TD children acting with a given vitality form, ASD children could not match the sensory representation of the observed action kinematics onto their own processes and representations of the corresponding vitality form. The same happens with neurotypical adults when observing ASD children acting with a given vitality form.

Taking the findings of all the above-mentioned studies into consideration leads us to suggest that the ability to understand the vitality forms of actions performed by other people is different to, and to a great extent independent of, the ability to understand their goal-directed actions, because it involves sensorimotor transformations of a different kind. We have already mentioned that the study of vitality forms is still in the early phases and there is no doubt that much still has to be done in order to have a clearer picture of the mirror property of the dorso-central portion of the insula. That said, these first studies seem to indicate that our claim that the sensorimotor transformations induced by DCI mirror responses play an important role in understanding the vitality forms expressed by others is more than plausible.

The Chapter in Brief

In this chapter we have claimed that mirror responses play a distinctive role in understanding other people's actions, emotions, and vitality forms.

Regarding actions, the mirror responses of the parieto-frontal areas trigger a transformation of the sensory representations concerning the observed actions into the motor processes and representations that are typically recruited when those actions are executed rather than being observed. According to our claim, if observing someone execute a particular action results in the recruitment of motor processes and representations similar to those that would come into play were the observer to plan for and execute that action themselves, this recruitment will enable them to identify the goal(s) of the observed action. This means that how people identify the goal(s) of an action they are observing may depend on how they represent the action motorically. If their motor representation of the action goal(s) changes, all things being equal their understanding of that action when observing it rather than executing it will change also. This is our claim, and in this chapter (pp. 155–190) we have seen that there are four distinct lines of evidence to support it.

This also holds true for emotions such as disgust and fear. The mirror responses of the anterior portion of the insula and the amygdala trigger a transformation of the visual representations regarding the facial (and bodily) expressions of disgust or fear we observe in others, into the visceromotor processes and representations typically recruited when we experience those emotions ourselves. Once again, our claim is that if seeing someone grimacing in disgust or fear results in the recruitment of visceromotor processes and representations similar to those that would be recruited were we ourselves to experience these emotions, it allows us to identify them and recognize that they are indeed expressive of disgust or fear. In our view, how we recognize the kind of emotion another person is displaying may depend on how we represent that kind of emotion and how these representations shape our own experience of it. If the visceromotor representation of an emotion and its corresponding experience are damaged in some way, the understanding of that emotion when observed in others will also be affected. The studies conducted on patients suffering from lesions of the anterior insula or the amygdala cited in this chapter (pp. 193–202) show that this is indeed the case.

Last but not least, we have extended our claim to include Daniel Stern's vitality forms. We have seen that observing actions executed with a particular vitality form elicits a mirror response from the dorso-central portion of the insula, which in turn triggers a transformation of the sensory representations regarding the action being observed into the motor processes and representations that are involved when that action is executed with that vitality form, as opposed to being observed. In this case, if observing an action executed with a particular vitality form recruits motor processes and representations similar to those we would call into play if we were to plan and execute that action ourselves, then this recruitment enables us to identify the vitality form and recognize that it characterizes the action we are observing. Although research on vitality forms is still in the early stages, the findings from the studies reviewed in this chapter (pp. 203–213) appear to provide evidence in favour of our claim.

CHAPTER 6

UNDERSTANDING FROM THE INSIDE

In this final chapter we will provide a brief recap of the main claims concerning the mirror property and the mirror mechanism that we introduced and discussed in the preceding chapters. The *first claim* relates to the finding that the mirror mechanism characterizes a large number of functionally different brain structures; this motivates considering this mechanism as a fundamental principle of the functional organization of the nervous system (Chapter 1). The *second claim* is that mirror responses involve sensorimotor or sensori-visceromotor transformations that are specifically related to different kinds of action goals, emotions, or vitality forms (Chapters 2, 3, and 4). And it is due to these transformations, according to the *third claim*, that mirror responses may play a distinctive role in understanding the actions, emotions, and vitality forms of other people (Chapter 5).

The first two claims relate to the anatomical and functional characteristics of neurons possessing the mirror property and to the kind of processes and representations that the various mirror responses can trigger. The third claim differs in nature, in that it concerns the possibility that the processes and representations

Mirroring Brains. Giacomo Rizzolatti and Corrado Sinigaglia, Oxford University Press. © Oxford University Press 2023. DOI: 10.1093/oso/9780198871705.003.0006

evoked by mirror responses contribute specifically to the capability of understanding what other people are doing or feeling.

Despite years of accumulating evidence in support of this last claim, as we have already mentioned, it is still being debated. This, however, is hardly surprising, for at least two reasons. The first is *experimental* in nature and has its roots in the difficulty of integrating measures and data obtained with techniques and procedures that are by no means homogeneous. The second is *conceptual* and pertains to the fact that 'understanding', like expressions such as 'knowing' and 'intending', are often used with various meanings in both everyday language and specialist literature.

In the following pages we will try to clarify what we mean when we write about 'understanding' other people's actions, emotions, and vitality forms. We will also try to demonstrate that the findings presented and discussed in the preceding chapters support the attribution to mirror neurons of a distinctive role in our capability of grasping and judging what we see other people doing. This will provide us with the opportunity both to reply to objections that have been raised against our (third) claim, and also to argue that this claim implicates, among other things, that the experiences we acquire while observing other people's actions and emotions are in certain respects similar to our own experiences when executing those actions or living those emotions ourselves.

Identifying Goals

So, when we speak about understanding other people's actions, what do we mean exactly? The first answer that comes to mind, and maybe the most natural, is that whoever is watching the action has some knowledge concerning the beliefs, desires, and intentions of the observed agent and this knowledge reveals the reasons for their action. This is not only close to the commonly accepted sense of the verb 'to understand' but also, whether consciously or unconsciously, adheres to a longstanding philosophical tradition whereby an action is a behaviour rationally motivated by beliefs, desires, and intentions.[1] These are the agent's mental states that identify the intentional content of an action, thereby not only differentiating it from actions of a different kind but also from the mere sequence of physical movements that constitutes it. If an action is the action that it is in virtue of its relation to an agent's beliefs, desires, and intentions, understanding that action means grasping how the action is linked to the agent's mental states.

If we take a closer look at the commonly accepted meaning of 'understanding', however, we can see that it does not rule out the possibility of talking about having understood an observed action without necessarily possessing any knowledge of the mental states that might have provided the agent with reasons for executing it. Let's take an example to illustrate this: imagine seeing a person reaching for a glass. Someone asks you if you have understood what that person is doing. Your answer might reasonably be, 'Yes, of course, they are going to pick up that glass'. You might even say, 'They are going to pick up the glass to drink from it' or 'They are going to pick up the glass to put it in the sink'. Your answers could be appropriate even if you have no knowledge about the mental states that motivated the person to reach for the glass. In this case, understanding the observed action means representing one or

---

[1] Here, and in the following pages, we have used the concepts of belief, desire, and intention in the pretheoretical sense typical of folk psychology in order to be as neutral as possible vis-à-vis the various notions found in literature.

more potential action goals (e.g. picking up the glass, picking up the glass to drink from it, or picking up the glass to put it in the sink) and identifying which of these are among the actual goals (picking up the glass to drink from it rather than picking up the glass to put it in the sink, say) of the observed action.[2] Identification of the actual action goal can lead the observer to try to fathom the mental states they suppose might have motivated the agent to execute that action directed at that particular goal, of course. However, goal identification does not in itself presuppose such knowledge.[3]

In the following pages we will use the phrase *full-blown understanding of the action* to avoid any possible ambiguity when the term 'understanding' involves (among other things) knowledge of the mental states that supposedly motivated the agent to perform the action, and *basic understanding of the action* when the observer identifies the actual action goal(s) without this necessarily involving any degree of knowledge of the mental states that led to the action being executed.[4]

---

[2] Here, as in Chapter 2 (p. 00), we are using the term *goal* in the sense of an actual or possible outcome of an action. Indeed, this is the most commonly accepted sense of the term: for example, we would say that 'our goal is to write as good a book as we can'. Similarly, when we talk about identifying goals, we refer to the outcomes that we expect the actions we are observing to have if things go well for the agent, rather than the states of the agent executing the actions. By contrast, *goal representations* are the states, generally of intentions, beliefs or desires that represent the outcome of an action and by virtue of which the action can be directed to that outcome.

[3] See Allen (2010) on this topic, while Goldman (2006) is obligatory reading for an in-depth discussion of the different forms of understanding, particularly in relation to the processes and representations evoked by mirror responses (see also Goldman (2009)). See also Gallese, Sinigaglia (2011), Sinigaglia, Butterfill (2015a), and Rizzolatti, Sinigaglia (2016).

[4] It could be objected that while this distinction does have some legitimacy given the vagueness of the commonly accepted meaning of the term *understand*, its usefulness is only apparent, since (hence the objection) we cannot understand

The studies and findings examined in Chapters 2 and 4 indicate that the basic understanding of an observed action can depend decisively on the processes and representations induced by mirror responses. In Chapter 2 we saw that:

- mirror responses while observing people executing actions can involve a transformation, in the observer, of the sensory representations regarding these actions into motor representations of one or more action goals, such as *picking up an object, kicking something,* but also *playing a chord on a musical instrument, executing a dance* or *a capoeira step,* and so on;
- these representations can trigger processes in the observer that are similar to those recruited while planning and executing actions with these kinds of action goals.

For this reason, observing an action can influence the execution of that kind of action and vice versa (Brass et al., 2000; Kilner et al., 2003; Craighero et al., 2002). This is also why, when we observe an action, we are not only able to represent its goal(s) motorically, but also to understand the action itself by identifying its actual goal(s). This can enable an observer to *anticipate* with their gaze the outcome to which the observed action is directed. As we saw in Chapter 5, the mirror response is *sufficient,* all things being equal, to guarantee that this anticipation of the outcome is timely and,

the goal of an action without knowing something about what the agent who is executing that action believes they are doing, or desires or intends to do. As we will see in the following pages, there are a number of well-founded considerations against this objection. Of these, first and foremost, is the fact that the representation of a goal is not, or is not exclusively, a matter of beliefs, desires, and intentions. As we saw in Chapter 2, goals can also be represented motorically. See Butterfill and Sinigaglia (2014) for a detailed discussion of this point.

above all, accurate (Flanagan & Johanson, 2003; Ambrosini et al., 2011). In fact, if during the observation of an action we are unable, even temporarily, to represent its goal motorically, the timeliness and accuracy of anticipatory gaze will be lost (Costantini, Ambrosini, Cardellicchio et al., 2014).

In Chapter 5, we saw that mirror responses can also influence our capability of *judging* actual action goal(s) (Cattaneo et al., 2011). It is important to keep in mind that this influence is *content-specific*, in the sense that our judgement varies according to the different motor representations evoked. Indeed, the cases we reviewed in the last chapter regarding perceptual judgements of the physical properties of an object (Hamilton et al., 2004; Jacobs & Shiffrar, 2005; Pobric & Hamilton, 2006), perceived direction of movement (Wohlschläger, 2000), apparent motion paths (Shiffrar & Freyd, 1990; Stevens et al., 2000), and the pitch height of a sequence of tones (Repp & Knoblich, 2007), also support the hypothesis that this judgement will be content-specific for the processes and motor representations of the observer. This would explain why an increase in motor expertise, among other things, produces a facilitation effect and an increase in the timeliness and accuracy of the judgement regarding observed action goals, and why this effect is selective for the actions for which we have developed a specific motor expertise (Aglioti et al., 2008; Shiffrar & Heinen, 2011).

Mirror responses and a Full-Blown Understanding of Action

Earlier we distinguished between a *basic* and *full-blown understanding* of an action. Full-blown understanding requires knowledge of the agent's mental states and using this knowledge in order to either explain why the agent performed the action or to predict its occurrence. The findings discussed in Chapter 5 indicate that mirror responses play a critical role in identifying the goals of the observed actions, impacting on how those actions are perceptually judged. Is there any evidence that the mirror responses and their corresponding sensorimotor transformations can also play a role in full-blown understanding of action?

Studies conducted up till now have not thrown much light on this subject. Marcel Brass and colleagues applied functional brain imaging to a group of participants while they were watching video clips of an unusual action being executed in plausible and implausible contexts (Brass et al., 2007). In one of the clips, a girl is seen to be operating a light switch with her right knee while her hands are (a) free, (b) partially occupied and (c) fully occupied. On an independent behavioural test, condition (a) was considered to be less plausible than (b), which in turn was judged to be less plausible than (c). If you see someone switching on a light or opening a door with their knee, you would consider it to be normal behaviour if their hands are occupied, but not if their hands are free or could be freed to execute the action. The analysis of the BOLD signal in the contrast between conditions (a) – (c) and (b) – (c), picked up differential activation in the posterior portion of the STS and in the anterior portion of the median frontal cortex. No differential activation was found in the parieto-frontal areas that are classically known to have the mirror property.

Roman Liepelt and colleagues at the Max Planck Institute in Leipzig obtained similar results from an fMRI study in which the participants were asked to observe finger movements in four different conditions: in the first, the fingers were raised naturally (*standard movement*); in the second, they were raised by a wire (*passive movement*); in the third, the raised fingers were closed in a clamp so movement was very limited (*restrained movement*), and in the fourth, the finger movement was minimal (*micro movement*) (Liepelt et al., 2008). The comparison of the various conditions showed that observing finger micromovements when no external restrictions to movement had been applied resulted in an activation in the right hemisphere of the posterior portion of the STS and particularly of the so-called temporo-parietal junction. No differential activation was found in the brain areas known to possess the mirror property, except between the active and passive movements.

How should we interpret these data? According to the authors, both studies show that when actions are executed in an unusual manner or in a way that the participants do not find immediately plausible, the mirror response is integrated with an inferential process that allows the observer to capitalize on the relevant contextual information in order to figure out the agent's states, which could provide an indication as to why the action was executed in this or that way (see Brass et al., 2007, p. 2120; Liepelt et al., 2008, p. 791). This interpretation seems to be corroborated by an fMRI study carried out by Floris de Lange and colleagues at the University of Nijmegen, in which the participants were presented with a number of common everyday actions such as picking up a cup, which could however be executed with uncommon goals such as lifting the cup to an ear, or in an unusual manner such as grasping the cup from above by its rim and lifting it to the mouth. In certain trials they were asked just to watch the actions, while in others they had to judge whether the action had an unusual goal or had been executed in an unusual manner. The authors found that when the participants just watched the actions, including those with an unusual goal, there was an increase in the activity of the inferior frontal gyrus, an area which is known to possess the mirror property; on the other hand, when they were asked to judge whether the goal was common or unusual, there was an increase in the activity of the posterior portion of the right STS, of the posterior sector of the cingulate cortex, and the prefrontal mesial cortex (de Lange et al., 2008).

As a result, some researchers have hypothesized a 'division of labour': mirror responses and their corresponding transformations are primarily involved in action goal recognition while a network of areas including the posterior portion of the STS and the TPJ are primarily involved in acquiring knowledge about the person's beliefs, desires, and intentions (Kilner & Frith, 2007; Keysers & Gazzola, 2007). Without getting entangled in the *vexata quaestio* of the existence of a network of areas specifically dedicated to reading other minds (see Saxe et al., 2004, among others), we must point out that these studies did not include tasks requiring the participants to represent explicitly, and in a controlled manner, the mental states of other persons as a motivating reason for their action. It is true that observing unusual or somewhat unlikely actions might induce the observer to infer the reasons behind such behaviour, but this does not automatically mean that they will infer the mental states that caused the agent to behave as they did. If the car in front of you at the traffic lights does not immediately start when the lights change to green, you may think the driver is a beginner or that their car has a mechanical problem. Of course, you might think that the driver *believes* it is better to wait a moment before proceeding, but our experience on the road indicates that few drivers actually think like this.

In point of fact, in the studies conducted by Brass and Liepelt the observed actions had the *same goal*, e.g. pressing a switch or raising a finger. What changed was the *way* in which the goal was achieved. If we reflect on what we have seen in the preceding chapters, it comes as no surprise that there was no *differential* activation of the mirror areas when comparing these conditions. Quite the contrary, given that the data we presented and discussed in Chapters 2 and 5 clearly indicate that mirror responses can relate to the observed action goal independently of the manner in which it is achieved. *Additional* activation when comparing unusual or unlikely conditions in areas such as the posterior portion of the STS or TPJ is not necessarily an indicator of a mindreading process, attributing people being observed with states that would provide motivating reasons for their ways of performing actions, as indeed the authors themselves admit. It must also be remembered that the role of the TPJ is still being debated, starting from the distinction between a more anterior sector, which is also involved in reorienting attention (see Corbetta et al., 2008 among others) and a more posterior sector, which some authors (Saxe & Kanwisher, 2003) suggest specializes in attributing mental states while several studies report activation of the most posterior sector of the TPJ in tasks which did not imply any mind reading in spite of having certain social connotations (for example, see Cook et al., 2014; Sowden & Catmur, 2015; Bardi et al., 2017). It must also be remembered that the posterior sector of the right STS is known to be involved in the representation of biological movements executed with the hands or other body parts; although this representation can contribute to some degree to the attribution of mental states such as beliefs and intentions (Frith & Frith, 2003), it is not in itself sufficient to provide a full-blown understanding of the action.

This does not mean that it is impossible to investigate whether, and if so to what extent, mirror responses contribute to the full-blown understanding of observed actions. Quite the opposite, in fact. The discussion of the studies we have reviewed earlier could suggest a different approach. Instead of focusing on a 'division of labour', it would be much more interesting to explore whether the way in which action goals are represented motorically may have a content-specific effect on how mental states such as beliefs or intentions are represented and, if this is so, to what extent. Just as an example, a study could be conducted to investigate whether an increase in motor expertise could have an impact on the observer's capability to explain the action being observed in terms of the agent's mental states, regardless of whether the outcome is positive or negative. Along similar lines, it would also be interesting to explore the effect and degree of interference caused by electromagnetic stimulation or lesions to the parieto-frontal regions possessing the mirror property in accurately and promptly representing mental states which may provide a person with the reasons for executing the observed actions. And, of course, the inverse also holds true. Indeed it would be extremely interesting to measure the effect that the attribution of mental states could have on mirror responses. In other words, mirror responses should be measured with tasks that vary the involvement of mindreading, in particular attributing (false) beliefs. In our view, regardless of the differences between the formats of the motor or visceromotor representations involved in the mirror responses and those of the representations and processes that characterize beliefs, desires, and intentions which have (or could have) propositional content, there could still nevertheless be cases in which what we give credence to about the beliefs, desires, and intentions of other people depends, at least partially, on our capability of represent the goal(s) of the observed actions motorically.[5]

Understanding the Emotions of Others

Up to now we have focused on the domain of actions, but our claim is that mirror responses can also play a distinctive role in understanding other people's emotions. What exactly does this mean? The distinction between *basic* and *full-blown understanding* that we drew for actions can also be applied to the emotions.

A concrete example will help to clarify this concept. Imagine that you are travelling by train, and the person in the seat in front of you widens their eyes and lets their mouth drop open for a split second. Maybe this troubles you, but only for a moment; you go back to your book, dismissing the episode as having little or no importance. But maybe not; you might start wondering what caused the person to react that way. So you can hypothesize that maybe they saw or read something that made a particular impression on them or reminded them of an unpleasant experience from which they have not completely recovered. Or maybe this person is just easily upset, and so on. After a minute or so, you give in to temptation and start talking to the person, looking to create an opportunity to ask a question that will explain that momentary reaction.

---

[5] For further reading on the notion of representational formats and the challenge of explaining non-accidental harmonies among representations with different formats such as motor representations on the one hand and beliefs or intentions on the other, we recommend Butterfill and Sinigaglia (2014), Sinigaglia and Butterfill (2015a, 2015b).

Now, suppose someone asks you to pinpoint the *exact moment* you understood what the person sitting in front of you was feeling. Maybe you will reply that you understood immediately when you saw an expression of what was probably fear on their face. Or maybe you will say that you only understood it when you became aware of what could have evoked the reaction, of what the person thought and felt, of their state of mind, their character and so on, in brief everything that could explain what seemed to be a momentary flash of fear. Both replies are legitimate, reflecting the ambiguous meaning of the verb *to understand* of which we wrote earlier. To avoid this ambiguity, we will talk about *basic understanding* of other people's emotions when we are in a position to identify the kind of emotion being felt by another person without necessarily being aware of the circumstances that have provoked it or knowing the person involved. We will talk about *full-blown understanding* of other people's emotions when we are able not only to identify the kind of emotion being felt by the other person, but also to explain why that person, given their particular character, state of mind, sensibilities, and beliefs, experienced that kind of emotion in that particular situation and reacted in that particular way.[6]

In Chapters 3 and 5 we reviewed and discussed the finding that the mirror responses and corresponding sensori-visceromotor transformations can contribute critically to a *basic understanding* of other people's emotions. In fact, we know that:

– when observing someone else expressing emotions such disgust and fear, the mirror responses involve the transformation

---

[6] See Goldie (2000, pp. 181–189) for a similar distinction.

of the sensory representations regarding the expressions observed into the corresponding visceromotor representations; these representations trigger a series of vegetative and motor processes, similar to those that would be triggered were the observer themselves experiencing those kinds of emotion.

This is not to say that we need to have the same emotional reaction as the people we are observing in order to have a *basic understanding* of the emotion they are experiencing, as happens in cases of *emotional contagion*. You don't need to retch or grimace in disgust to understand that the person sitting across the table is revolted by the taste or the smell of the food they have been served; as long as your observation of the other person's disgust elicits visceromotor processes and representations *similar* to those that are evoked when you yourself are exposed to that food, you will understand their emotional reaction. In fact, all things being equal, these are the processes and representations that allow us, as observers, to link the observed expressions to the corresponding emotions.

In Chapter 5 we also saw that mirror responses can influence how people judge the kind of emotion another person is experiencing. Take the cases of N.K. and B., the patients with lesions in the AI (pp. 193–194). They scored below normal on tasks involving recognition of expressions of disgust both when these involved observing grimaces when tasting foul food or listening to sounds similar to retching, while their performances were within the norm when another kind of facial expression, such as joy or fear, was involved. These patients did not show a deficit in visual recognition of faces, nor did they have any difficulty in understanding the concepts of the various emotions, disgust included. In other words, they were perfectly aware of the meaning of the term 'disgust' and what can evoke it, but they were unable to respond appropriately to stimuli soliciting disgust or disgusting situations; indeed, in more than one test they were seen to have a deficit in the experience of disgust (Calder et al., 2000; Adolphs et al., 2003). Their difficulty in representing disgust visceromotorically not only affected their capability to react to unpleasant smells, revolting foodstuffs, and the experiences that these reactions could provoke, it also negatively affected their capability of recognizing other people's experiences of disgust. Similar difficulties in disgust recognition have been induced by direct electric stimulation of the AI (Papagno et al., 2016); the transient inactivation of the AI temporarily blocked the observer from recruiting the visceromotor representations that were typically involved in their own experience of disgust.

The same holds true for fear. Studies conducted with patients suffering from lesions of the amygdala have shown an association between the existence of a deficit in the capability of representing fear visceromotorically and thereby to experience it personally, and the capability of recognizing fear when experienced by other individuals (pp. 198–201). A case in point is that of S.M., studied for many years by Ralph Adolphs and his collaborators. Although S.M. knew what fear is and how to behave in potentially dangerous situations, she had difficulty in putting this into action and was unable to feel fear in situations that other people found extremely frightening (Adolphs et al., 1994; Adolphs et al., 1995; Adolphs et al., 1999). Moreover, her visceral and physiological reactions to potentially dangerous stimuli were very different from those of the controls (Bechara et al., 1995). These difficulties were accompanied by a clear deficit in understanding other people's experience of fear: she tended systematically to underestimate it; she was unable to imitate facial expressions of fear and was not even able to sketch frightened faces.

This all goes to suggest that mirror responses can determine a basic understanding of other people's emotions, influencing the capability of the observer to judge the kind of emotion another person is experiencing. Taking these distinctions into consideration, the question that naturally comes to mind is whether there is evidence that mirror responses and visceromotor transformations play a role in what we have called *full-blown understanding* of other people's emotions.

Although a number of studies have attempted a systematic investigation of the cerebral areas specifically involved in mindreading tasks with a clear emotional valence (see Shamay-Tsoory, 2011, for a review), we know little or nothing about if and how mirror responses can contribute, even partially, to a full-blown understanding of other people's emotions. That said, we can go back to what has already been suggested in the case of actions with no emotional valence. One way of dealing with this issue could be to see whether, and if so to what extent, differences in the capability of representing emotions such as disgust and fear visceromotorically could affect the capability of accounting for those emotions when they are experienced by others. There are studies in which recruitment of visceromotor processes and representations biases perceptual judgements of the category or intensity of a facially expressed emotion—particularly when the manner in which the face is presented is ambiguous (see Niedenthal et al., 2010; Naor et al., 2018, among others). This bias effect could be investigated further, to see whether and to what extent it is present in affective mindreading tasks. It would also be worthwhile to explore whether mirror responses could be influenced by the observer executing explicit affective mindreading tasks. Our hypothesis for emotions, as for actions, is that although the processes and representations called into play by mirror responses differ in format from the representations and processes involved in affective mindreading, there can still be cases in which what the observer thinks about the emotional states of other people depends, at least partially, on their capacity to visceromotorically represent the emotional expressions they are observing.

Understanding other People's Vitality Forms

Vitality forms, which as we have seen characterize the dynamics of actions and emotions, constitute one of the areas of greatest interest in the study of the various modalities of understanding. In the previous chapters we saw that more than one study has found mirror responses, at least those regarding action-related vitality forms, in the dorso-central portion of the insula (DCI) (Di Cesare et al., 2015; Di Cesare, Fasano, Errante et al., 2016; Di Cesare et al., 2018). In addition, we have introduced and discussed the claim that DCI mirror responses and the corresponding sensorimotor transformations play a distinctive role in understanding the vitality forms characteristic of observed actions (pp. 203–213). The distinctions explained in the preceding pages help to clarify the nature of this understanding. In this regard, it is important to keep in mind that:

– while we are observing actions executed with a particular vitality form (e.g. gentle or rude), DCI mirror responses entail the transformation of the sensory representations concerning the observed actions into the corresponding motor representations;

– these representations elicit in the observer a series of processes similar to those that would be called into play if instead of observing the action, they themselves were to execute it with that same kind of vitality form.

If in fact this is the case, DCI mirror responses and their corresponding sensorimotor transformations allow the observer to represent the form (*how*) of an action, regardless of its content (*what*). The following examples will help to clarify this: remember when you were particularly impressed by the sight of a *natural* or *forced* expression on someone's face, by a *courteous* gesture or a *rude* one, by *discreet* peal of laughter or a *coarse* guffaw? In many cases, you will have identified the expression, the gesture, or the laughter and will have been pleasantly (or unpleasantly) surprised. This is a very common experience, so common we tend to ignore it, but just think how difficult life would be if we were not able to capture the connection that turns the motion of the hand that we have just observed into a *fond* farewell or a *brusque* dismissal.

In Chapter 5 we reviewed data that appears, at least in this early phase, to suggest that DCI mirror responses can contribute critically to a *basic understanding* of action-related vitality forms, influencing the observer's capability of judging them. For example, Di Cesare and colleagues showed that when their participants were required to judge the vitality form of observed actions, a selective activation of the DCI ensued that was not present when they were asked to judge a physical property of those actions such as speed, in spite of the fact that the stimuli were exactly the same (Di Cesare et al., 2014; Di Cesare, Valente, Di Dio et al., 2016).

Research regarding basic understanding of other people's vitality forms is still in the preliminary phase, but we know even less about whether and how DCI responses can contribute to what we can call, drawing an analogy with the definition explained earlier, *full-blown understanding* of the vitality forms observed in others. This level of understanding not only requires identification of the kind of vitality forms that characterize the observed actions, but also knowledge of the reasons that induced them, which can also be sought in the agent's thoughts, feelings, or motivations. In fact, the state of full-blown understanding of other people's vitality forms has never been studied in an experimental format, nor are there yet any mindreading tasks designed specifically to investigate the attribution of mental states concerning the form or style of observed actions (or of emotional reactions).

We have mentioned many times that vitality forms in themselves are not reducible to either actions or emotions because they characterize the expressive dynamics of both. Therefore, if we are to investigate what kind of processes and representations might be involved in fully understanding the vitality forms of others, we need to design completely new experimental paradigms. Specifically, we need to create new experimental designs to assess whether, and if so to what extent, a full-blown understanding of the vitality forms of other people can be modulated by our own capability of representing these forms when we ourselves are executing the action or displaying the emotional reaction that we have observed in others. Our hypothesis is that, as we have seen for actions and emotions, mirror responses will in some way influence our thoughts regarding the mental states that may have led the agent we are observing to perform an action or to express an emotion with one kind of vitality form instead of another.

Objections and Responses

In the preceding pages we have attempted to clarify our claim that mirror responses play a distinctive role in understanding other people's actions, emotions, and vitality forms, which gives us the opportunity, among other things, to reply to a number of objections that have been raised against this claim over the years. Although most of these objections challenge our claim in the domain of actions, we will also use data from research regarding the domains of emotions and vitality forms in our rebuttal.

The *first objection* concerns the *characteristic traits* of mirror responses; to cut a long story short, the fact that they may exhibit different degrees of congruency between the executed and the observed actions could create a certain 'tension' regarding their alleged role in action understanding. In cases where there is a strong congruence, the motor representation would return a copy, so to speak, of the action being observed; the mirror response would benefit in accuracy, but would lose in terms of generality. On the other hand, if the congruence is broad, the motor representation of the action being observed is much less detailed and the mirror response would benefit in terms of generality but would not be so accurate (Csibra, 2007; Jacob, 2009). One might be tempted to conclude that the claim of a distinctive role for mirror responses in understanding action is not consistent with these differences in the degree of congruency; if the characteristic trait of the mirror responses consists—as the term itself would seem to indicate, at least at a first glance—in a very strict congruence between the visual and motor representations of the action, then the role that these responses could have in understanding action would be limited to a very restricted sphere of actions. On the other hand, if the broadly congruent responses were to be considered, for all intents and purposes, as being mirror responses, then the sphere of the actions involved would expand, but the extent to which the mirror responses could contribute to understanding the action would not be clear by any means, given the inaccuracy of the sensorimotor transformations involved. This is the first objection.

Although this line of reasoning is tempting, we think that there are good reasons to reject this objection. First of all, it must be remembered that the different degrees of congruency of the mirror responses mostly regard the representation of action *goals*. We have mentioned several times that the observer can motorically represent the outcome to which the action they are observing is directed with different degrees of generality. For example, the sight of a hand assuming a certain grip while moving towards an object of a given size can evoke in the observer motor representations of outcomes such as *grasping, grasping with a hand, grasping with a precision grip* (or a *whole hand*), and so on (Rizzolatti et al., 2001). Some of these representations can be strictly congruent, specifically representing the outcome of the action being observed; others have a broader degree of congruency, representing the same outcome in less detail, but still sufficient to distinguish it from other goals. Others again will represent the outcome differently depending on whether or not it is inserted in a complex architecture of goals.

In this, mirror responses are no different from the responses of the motor neurons that trigger the motor processes and representations involved in the short-term planning, execution, and control of the action. The outcome(s) of an action can be motorically represented with varying degrees of generality both in the observer and the person executing the action (Rizzolatti et al., 1988). In Chapter 2 we saw that there are neurons in the ventral premotor cortex (F5) of the macaque that respond identically when the animal grasps an object with its right hand, left hand or mouth (pp. 41–43) and that motor representations of a goal such as grasping could differ according to whether they are linked to another goal (pp. 44–45), such as lifting an object to the mouth or placing it in a container, independently of where the container is located (Fogassi et al., 2005). Regardless of whether we are executing the action personally or are observing it being executed, all such representations can contribute to motorically representing its outcome(s), triggering those processes that guarantee that the motorically represented outcome(s) constitute the goal(s) to which the action is directed.

Far from creating any 'tension', these different degrees of congruency of the mirror responses contribute to clarifying the specific role that they can play in action understanding. As we have seen, differences in motor expertise can result in a different measure of capability, not only in representing the observed action goals motorically but also in identifying and even judging them. Basketball, volleyball, and darts players, indeed experts in any kind of action, are generally quicker and more accurate in identifying the outcome of the actions they are observing when these fall within their area of expertise (pp. 166–178). The possibility of recruiting motor processes and representations is not in itself a guarantee that we will have a sufficient understanding of the action we are observing. Indeed, the more the processes and representations induced by observing an action are able to capture its goal(s) motorically, the better will be our understanding of the action we are observing. On the other hand, if our capability of motorically representing the goal(s) of the action we are observing is not very well-developed, as may be the case if we do not possess specific motor expertise in this action, then it will have less impact on our understanding of the action.[7] This is our reply to the *first* objection.

A *second* objection has been raised, which directly regards the possibility that mirror neurons play a specific role in understanding actions. In a nutshell, some authors claim that actions can be understood without any assistance from mirror responses (Hickok, 2009, 2014; Caramazza et al., 2014). This objection is usually supported by two arguments: the *first* insists on the notion that processes and representations other than those evoked by mirror responses can support the understanding of actions, while the *second* is based on a number of studies on patients suffering from apraxia and the possible dissociations they revealed between action execution and understanding.

With regard to the *first argument*, an fMRI study conducted by Giovanni Buccino and colleagues is frequently cited in the premises; these authors showed that observing an action with the goal of biting activated parieto-frontal areas in the observer that are known to have the mirror property, regardless of whether the biting was being done by a human, a monkey, or a dog. In contrast,

---

[7] The study conducted by Vasudevi Reddy et al. on anticipatory gaze and motor skills in infancy is relevant to this point. The authors showed how infants were able to anticipate the outcome of a perceived action as early as 6 months of age providing the action consisted in grasping an object with a whole-hand grasp. Proactive gazes when observing a grasping action executed with a precision grip were only found from 8 to 10 months of age. Of great interest is the fact that the rapidity and accuracy with which the infants anticipated the outcome of the observed action with their gaze, correlated with their capability of grasping different sized objects with increasing accuracy. In other words, the greater their capability of motorically representing the 'grasping' goal with different degrees of generality, evidenced by their capability in grasping and manipulating objects requiring different hand shapes, the more able they were to understand rapidly and accurately the actions that they were observing, regardless of the type of grasp used (Ambrosini et al., 2013; see also Cannon and Woodward, 2012).

watching a dog barking evoked activation of the observer's visual areas, but not the parieto-frontal mirror areas. These did activate however when the agent was a human (Buccino et al., 2004).

It is of course hardly surprising that the mirror neurons did not discharge when the participants watched the dog barking; barking is not an action belonging to the human motor repertoire so no sensorimotor transformation was possible. However, the fact that humans are not able to represent barking motorically does not in itself exclude the possibility of understanding what the dog is doing, as the authors themselves acknowledge. Indeed, this is the case in many kinds of action: consider for a moment the flight of birds or bats, the slithering of snakes. When all is said and done, it is much the same for actions that belong to the human motor repertoire, but not to that of a specific individual, such as a move in Tai Chi for someone who has never practised martial arts or playing a cord on a violin for someone who has no expertise in playing this instrument. In both these cases, it is possible for the observer to somehow understand the action, or at least part of it, without calling on the mirror responses and their corresponding sensorimotor transformations. But this does not constitute a problem for our claim (contra Hickok, 2009, p. 5).

Claiming that mirror responses play a distinctive role in understanding action does not mean that they are *necessary* for understanding all kinds of action. According to our hypothesis, all things being equal, mirror responses are *sufficient* for something like a basic understanding of an observed action and can exert a content-respecting influence on what the observer *thinks* of the action, so putting them in a condition to judge it with greater accuracy. This of course does not rule out the possibility for the observer to understand the observed action by capitalizing on different kinds of processes or representations, such as inferential processes based on sensory representations.

Furthermore, there are at least two reasons why the fact that higher-order visual responses can be relevant for action understanding is certainly not an issue for our claim. The first is that the fact that the observation of an action elicits selective visual responses in higher-order areas such as the STS is perfectly compatible with this claim. Indeed, in Chapter 2 we discussed the seminal work by Perrett and colleagues in which the authors demonstrated that these responses can represent a wide variety of actions (Perrett et al., 1985; Perrett et al., 1989). All the same, and this is the second reason, the fact that the observed actions can be represented in higher-order visual areas such as the STS in no way implies that mirror responses have no role to play in the representation of an observed action, nor that they are unimportant for the observer's capacity to individuate observed action goals.

In Chapter 2, we also explained how the mirror neurons in the parieto-frontal areas (PFG/AIP and F5) can represent the observed action goal in such a degree as not to modify their response profile even when the action is executed with different effectors (the mouth as opposed to the hand, etc.) or even with a tool such as normal pliers or reverse pliers (these latter requiring opposite movements compared to the standard version) (Rizzolatti et al., 2001; Rochat et al., 2010). This does not apply to the visual responses of the STS as Luigi Cattaneo and colleagues demonstrated; STS responses are effector-specific, representing the observed actions on the basis of the body parts involved (Cattaneo et al., 2010) unlike the parieto-frontal mirror responses that can represent action goals even when these are realized with different effectors. This difference in goal representation is also reflected in the difference of their contributions towards understanding the observed action. More than one of the studies we reviewed in Chapter 5 have shown how, all things being equal, the possibility of relying on the mirror responses and their corresponding sensorimotor transformations has a significant impact on the understanding of the observed action, speeding it up and improving its accuracy. For example, Marcello Costantini and colleagues showed that although repetitive stimulation of the pSTS did have a certain effect on gaze proactivity, it was extremely diminished and unspecific compared to stimulation of the PMv, which drastically reduced the capability of the observer to anticipate the outcome of the observed action (Costantini, Ambrosini, Cardellicchio et al., 2014).

As clearly indicated by the above, the possibility of mirror responses playing a distinctive role in understanding the actions of others is in no way invalidated by the fact that such an understanding sometimes relies on sources other than the motor processes and representations of the person observing the action, nor by the fact that processing higher-order sensory representations may involve cortical structures such as the STS. Quite the opposite. Indeed, the very fact that an action can be understood in the absence of mirror responses helps to improve our comprehension of what is so special about the mirror mechanism and how it contributes to the understanding of the actions of others.

We will discuss this point further later in the chapter, but before doing so, we will examine the *second argument* regarding the possibility of a dissociation between action execution and action understanding that emerged from studies on patients suffering from apraxia, which has thrown doubt on the possible role of the mirror mechanism in understanding action (Hickok, 2009).

In replying to this objection, we cannot help but point out that, as everyone with experience of clinical neuropsychology knows, identifying a patient by syndromic diagnosis is by definition different from identifying them on the basis of lesional criteria. In fact, although there has been a wide consensus regarding the identification criteria for the various forms of apraxia for some time now (De Renzi & Faglioni, 1999; Heilman et al., 1982), it is still far from clear which anatomic substrates are involved and in what way they contribute to the various apraxic deficits.[8] In classical literature, symptomatology ascribes the apraxic deficit to a difficulty in eliciting instructed actions, even when patients are able to spontaneously execute those actions in everyday life (Liepmann, 1900). It is hardly surprising therefore that many of these patients do not show a deficit in understanding actions carried out by other individuals. In fact, unless they are suffering from larger lesions involving other motor structures such as the parieto-frontal areas, they do not present deficits in the motor representation of possible action goals. The fact that they are able to understand actions they see other people executing is therefore perfectly compatible with our claim, which in any case does not imply that a deficit in executing an action invariably results in a deficit in the understanding

[8]   For example, apraxic disorders have been observed not only in patients with lesions of the inferior parietal lobe (Buxbaum et al., 2007) but also in patients with temporal and subcortical lesions (Tessari et al., 2007). Laurel Buxbaum et al. of the Moss Rehabilitation Research Institute in Pennsylvania recently conducted a prospective study of cerebral lesions with over seventy apraxic patients, using tool-related and pantomime gesture tasks and the imitation of meaningless actions. They found that deficits in all three tasks correlated with lesions in the posterior temporal and inferior parietal regions, with a prevalence of lesions in the inferior and medial posterior temporal regions for actions involving tools, and parietal lesions for what the authors called novel actions (Buxbaum et al., 2014). See Goldenberg (2014) for a discussion of these data.

of those actions (Rizzolatti et al., 2014). If anything, it is interesting to note that there are patients suffering from apraxia who, as well as presenting deficits in executing certain kinds of action, also have difficulty in identifying them (see Heilman et al., 1982; Rothi et al., 1985). According to our claim, it is to be expected that this association is consequent on lesions of areas possessing the mirror property. Indeed, this is what Pazzaglia and colleagues found in the two studies cited in the previous chapter (pp. 188–189). The first study showed how apraxic patients with lesions of the parieto-frontal areas overall presented a deficit in understanding the actions of others; this deficit was even more noticeable when the areas that are typically involved in the planning and execution of actions were affected by a lesion (Pazzaglia, Pizzamiglio, Pes et al., 2008). In the second study, the authors showed that in apraxic patients with lesions of the parieto-frontal areas, deficits in understanding actions executed with the hand or mouth were associated with disorders of the motor representation of those actions (Pazzaglia, Smania, Corato et al., 2008).[9]

So neither the *first* nor the *second objection* appears to provide sufficient grounds to abandon our thesis. However, there is a *third objection* still to be considered. Like the second, its aim is to throw doubt on the possibility that mirror responses can play a distinctive role

[9] The observation that some brain-damaged patients with lesions in the parieto-frontal areas were able to understand the actions they were watching cannot be considered as an objection to our claim (Hickok, 2009). Not only are Pazzaglia's data solid, it is perfectly normal for studies on a large patient sample to have individual differences, partly due to the fact that lesion sites rarely superimpose and partly because different people compensate for their lesions in different ways. One of the major challenges of the future for neuropsychology will be to recruit increasingly large patient samples so as to reduce the impact of individual differences (Adolphs, 2016).

in understanding action. This time, however, a different argument has been raised: the objection here is that mirror responses cannot play a distinctive role in understanding actions as this would presuppose the capability of applying a 'semantics' (Hickok, 2009, 2014), to master more or less 'abstract concepts' (Caramazza et al., 2014) and none of this could be imputed to the sensorimotor (sensori-visceromotor) transformations potentially induced by observing other people's actions or emotional expressions.

How can we refute this objection? Assuming the notion of concept to be sufficiently narrow, one line of defence could be to point out that there are cases of a basic understanding of action that do not presuppose the use of concepts; moreover, these are cases in which motor processes and representations play a relevant role. We could quote numerous studies here to show, for example, that the capability of infants to identify goals of the actions they see being executed does not depend primarily on having this or that 'concept' but varies according to their motor competences (see Woodward & Gerson, 2014 for a review). We know that from six months of age, when infants start to show a certain capability in grasping objects, they are able to identify the action goals of others, such as hugging a teddy bear or grasping a ball (Woodward, 1998, 1999). But they can in fact do this earlier, if they develop adequate motor skills. Jessica Sommerville and colleagues investigated the capability of three-month old infants to understand the goal-directedness of observed actions using the classic habituation paradigm, which consisted in watching cartoons showing actions that differed in their goal or trajectory (Sommerville et al., 2005). Prior to the habituation task, half of the infants participating in the study took part in a brief motor training session during which they tried to grasp toys while wearing a mitten covered in Velcro hook-and-loop to facilitate the grip, while the remaining infants were required to merely watch another person grasping similar objects. The authors found that only the infants who had practised catching the toys during the training session showed surprise when the action goal in the cartoon was different to that to which they had been accustomed, but they did not show this reaction when the trajectory alone was different. The other infants, who had not participated in the training session, showed no surprise at all (see also Gerson & Woodward, 2014; Bakker et al., 2016). It is rather difficult to attribute the different capability shown by the two groups of infants in identifying the action goals they were shown to a different degree of mastery of more or less abstract concepts. More credible by far is the explanation that even a minimum degree of motor expertise gained from a few minutes of play with a Velcro-covered mitten will secure the possibility of understanding the observed action.

This objection can also be rebutted with another argument. Although the representations evoked by mirror responses in the domains of action, emotion and vitality forms do not presuppose the capability of mastering abstract concepts as they are motor or visceromotor representations, they can nevertheless exert a content-respecting influence on the capability of judging actions, emotions, or vitality forms in other people. In other words, what we *think* of the goals of actions that we see people executing can depend on how we represent those goals motorically, *almost* as if we ourselves were executing those actions. If, for some reason, there is a change in how these goals are represented motorically, then all things being equal, what we *think* when we see people executing actions directed at these goals will also change (pp. 162–165).

Imagine for a moment that you are in the country with a friend, walking along a road with no illumination. Suddenly, you see a set of point-lights moving about, but the configuration of these lights means nothing to either of you. At first glance, you don't take much notice, but then you start to worry a little as the set of point-lights seems to be moving towards you. You twig to the fact that it is a person, but you have no idea what they could be doing. When the lights come even closer, you realize that the person is moving their legs, but in a manner that means nothing to you as the movements are not compatible with the act of walking or other means of loco-motion such as pedalling. Mystery. But fortunately your friend is a biking fanatic and sometimes plays around with new ways of using his bicycle. For some time now he has been practising using his bike with a device that lets him pedal backwards instead of with the classical forward motion, so he actually moves the bike forward by pedalling backwards. Unlike you, he wasn't in the least concerned when he saw the lights moving towards you as he im-mediately recognized the pattern and the movement as a person on a bicycle, pedalling backwards instead of forwards. 'Well yes, of course,' he says, 'the person could have put a light on the bike too, but having put lights on his arms and legs, he was recognizable at a pinch. If you look closely, you'll see that he is indeed cycling, but he is moving the pedals backwards instead of forwards.' Given this explanation, you too recognize that the person who just passed you was on a bike and pedalling backwards.

Now both you and your friend understood, in one way or an-other, what this third person was doing, what his action goals were. But you did this in different ways. Your understanding is based above all on your friend's explanation. There is nothing strange about this. We often pick up knowledge about actions that we see being executed, by exploiting other people's knowledge. We do this every time we consult an expert. Sometimes, what the expert says changes what we originally thought about what we saw, and this is what happened in our story. Initially you thought that the set of point-lights was someone moving; then as you received more sensory information, this changed your perception to someone moving their legs; finally, on the basis of the information you received from your friend, you were able to fit all the pieces of the puzzle together and realize that what you were seeing was a person on a bike, moving forwards but pedalling backwards. There is nothing particularly mysterious in all this. In your friend's case, however, things went rather differently. He immediately recognized that the set of lights was nothing more or less than a person on a bicycle, pedalling backwards but moving forwards. This did not depend on a different perceptual capability or a different degree of mastery of abstract concepts. Nor had he experienced this scene before in any way. We can comfortably assume that this was the first time either of you had had an experience like this, just as we can exclude the possibility that your friend's visual or auditive abilities were different from yours. The only significant difference between you was that your friend possessed a certain motor expertise with bizarrely hacked bicycles while you did not. As a result, he was able to recruit certain processes and representations while observing the point-lights. Indeed, unlike you, he was able to represent the goal of the action motorically. Other things being equal, it is very likely that it was this capability that triggered his understanding of the action you both saw.

It could be objected that this thought example has been created *ad hoc* and that things go differently in the real world. But if we think back on what we have seen in the previous chapter we will see that our thought experiment isn't so very different from those conducted in reality; one example is the study run by Casile & Giese (2006) that brought to light the strong connection between the capability of planning and controlling the execution of a given action and the capability of understanding it when we see that action executed by others.

After all, even Bradford Mahon and Alfonso Caramazza recognized that the capability of representing an action goal motorically can contribute to the understanding of the action by emphasizing that 'motor information *colors* conceptual processing, enriches it, and provides it with a relational context' (Mahon & Caramazza, 2008, p. 68, *our italics*). To quote these authors again, 'What we know about the world depends also on interactions between 'abstract' conceptual content and the sensory and motor systems'. Sensorimotor transformations such as those induced by mirror responses would therefore have the function of 'rooting' conceptual representations 'in the rich sensory and motor content that mediates our physical interaction with the world' that surrounds us, others included (*ibidem*). This is why such transformations can influence the very way in which we judge the action being observed, and why, if our motor processes and representations are impaired, we will have difficulty in understanding observed actions even when our conceptual processes and representations are intact.

This is in fact the case of those patients with lesions of the parieto-frontal areas we mentioned earlier, for whom the difficulty of executing or imitating actions is associated with the difficulty of recognizing them when executed by other people (Pazzaglia, Pizzamiglio, Pes et al., 2008; Pazzaglia, Smania Corato et al., 2008). None of these patients showed any deficit in understanding abstract concepts regarding the various kinds of action; their difficulty in understanding the actions they were observing seemed rather to be attributable to an inability to transform the sensory representations of these actions into the corresponding motor representations. This also happens in understanding the emotions. We have frequently referred to the case of S.M., studied by Ralph Adolphs and his colleagues for many years. S.M. had no problem in understanding the meaning of concepts such as fear and was perfectly capable of explaining what to do in potentially dangerous situations. In spite of her mastery of the concept of fear, however, she was not able to experience fear as other people do, nor to have an appropriate understanding of other people's expressions of fear (Adolphs et al., 1994; Adolphs et al., 1995; Adolphs et al., 1999).

We can therefore conclude that the *third objection*, like the first two, does not raise any solid grounds against our claim that mirror responses play a distinctive role in understanding other people's actions and emotions. In the next pages we will attempt to further characterize the nature of this understanding, with a particular focus on what happens when it can rely on mirror responses and their corresponding sensorimotor or visceromotor transformations.

Understanding from the Inside

In presenting and defending our claim we have used a number of conceptual distinctions to clarify the degree to which mirror responses play a role in understanding other people's actions, emotions, and vitality forms. Now, regardless of whether this understanding be basic or full-blown, in no way does our thesis imply that the representations and processes induced by mirror responses are a necessary condition for understanding other people's actions and emotions. After all, for mirror responses to play a role in understanding other people's actions, emotions, and vitality forms, there has to be the capability of representing those actions, emotions, and vitality forms as if they were being executed, experienced, or shown personally. But there is no doubt at all that we are sometimes able to understand what we are not able to represent in motor and visceromotor terms. We can take advantage of a plethora of other processes and representations to obtain an understanding of what we see; for example, we can recruit a series of sensory representations, interlinked by associative processes. The association of these representations could then in some way trigger inferential processes such as those we use when reasoning about events or representations of events, or when we reach a decision.

The question, therefore, is not whether mirror responses are necessary for understanding (clearly they are not), but what difference their involvement makes. What is it that changes when the observer calls on the representations and processes they would recruit if they were to execute that action or experience that emotional reaction themselves? The findings we have reviewed in the previous chapter clearly show that when this happens, there is a significant increase in the *speed,* and above all in the *accuracy,* with which actions and emotions are understood. Frequently, the observer is able to understand what they are observing much better and much more rapidly, and the more complex the task, the greater the difference. Take a moment to think about what it means to have an immediate grasp of other people's fear, disgust, or mirth.[10] The same is true for vitality forms: think how important it is to be able to grasp immediately how welcome or unwelcome your visit is, judging by the warmth or coolness of your reception, the tenor of a smile, whether it is kind or cruel, and so on.[11] And lastly, when you are watching an action, think how important it is to be able to understand the goal(s) to which it is directed, and to be able to do this with the speed and accuracy needed to react promptly and appropriately, if a reaction is required.

On more than one occasion we have defined this kind of understanding of other people's actions, emotions, and vitality forms as *understanding from the inside*.[12] Now, we do not intend *from the inside* to be construed as an allusion to some more or less mysterious form of intrusion into another person's mind or soul; we are simply referring to a concept that was known before the discovery of mirror neurons. Take the domain of actions, for example; for

[10] See Peter Goldie, among others, on this point: 'The central idea was that this [the capability of communicating emotions] is an adaptation – it has survived in our species because of the selectional advantage it conferred to our ancestors of being able to communicate emotions to other members of the species. What is important here is that the survival of this trait presupposes that other members of the species had the capability for recognizing facial expression and so forth as being communicating of an emotion, and this capability too was an adaptation. Given this sort of evolutionary explanation of our capability for recognizing emotion in others, it is not surprising that this recognition can be achieved very quickly, and 'outwith' practical reasoning' (Goldie, 2000, p. 182).
[11] It is not surprising to see that more than one author has considered the capability of understanding vitality forms as a fundamental component of those forms of interaction characteristic of so-called 'primary intersubjectivity' (see, among others, Trevarthen, 1998; Rochat, 1999; Bråten, 1998).
[12] See, for example, Rizzolatti and Sinigaglia (2010), Sinigaglia and Rizzolatti (2011), Rizzolatti and Sinigaglia (2013), and Rizzolatti and Sinigaglia (2016).

some time now sport psychologists have been distinguishing between the representations an athlete may have when they imagine
watching their performance in the third person and those they
have when they imagine actually executing it in the first person
(see Mahoney & Avener, 1977). A practical example will help to
make this clearer: close your eyes for a second and try to imagine
an athlete on the starting blocks of the hundred-metre race in the
Olympics, before the starter begins the count-down procedure.
These are moments to which athletes dedicate the maximum con-
centration, and it is very likely that the athlete you are imagining
is mentally reviewing the sequence of movements they will soon
be implementing. As often happens with athletes (but also with
other categories), they will be so engrossed in imagining the movements to be executed that they will simulate some of these, moving
arms and legs into the best race posture. You and the athlete are
both imagining an action. Yours is an *external* imagination, so to
speak; you are *seeing* the moves of the athlete in your imagination.
The athlete's imagination, on the other hand, is *from the inside*; they
are imagining *executing* those movements as if they were really executing them and their involvement is so intense that they partially
manifest externally the movements that they are simulating in-
ternally in their brain.

These two forms of imagination are usually characterized respectively as *visual imagery* and *motor imagery*. *Imagining seeing* is
very similar to *actual seeing*; for example, we know that whether
a person imagines seeing an object or actually sees it, its appearance depends on its size and the distance from which it is seen
(Kosslyn, 1978, 1996). The same holds true for the time needed to
explore an object, which depends on the subjective dimension of
the object for the person seeing it, whether the seeing is real or

imagined (Kosslyn et al., 1978). In addition, imagining seeing and actual seeing can influence and modulate each other (Ishai & Sagi, 1995; Pearson et al., 2008). Finally, there is evidence that imagining seeing and actually seeing not only share a common neural substrate but also recruit similar cortical activation patterns (see Page et al., 2011, among others).

Similarly, *imagining executing* an action is similar in many ways to *actually executing* an action. The time it takes to imagine reaching an object is more or less the same as it takes to actually reach it (Decety et al., 1989; Decety, 1996; Jeannerod, 1994). Furthermore, in the case of grasping actions, if we want to execute an action such as grasping a cup by its handle and the handle is oriented in such a way as to make grasping it difficult, additional effort is needed not only to actually grasp but also to imagine doing so (Parsons, 1994; Frak et al., 2001). Imagining executing an action can also interfere selectively with its actual execution. Let's illustrate this with an example. There is a row of objects in front of you; imagine taking one. If immediately after, you are asked to actually take one of these objects but it is not the one you imagined taking, you will be slower than usual in executing the action (Ramsey et al., 2010). This interference comes as no surprise given that imagining executing an action and actually executing it involves similar parieto-frontal circuits and makes use of the same kind of motor processes and representations (Jeannerod & Decety, 1995; Jeannerod, 2001).

The *similarity* between imagining acting and actually acting and the *difference* between imagining acting and imagining seeing, provide the opportunity to elucidate a *first* characterization of the notion of understanding *from the inside*. You can imagine seeing a ball rotating on its axis but you cannot imagine rotating a ball or any other object 360 degrees, because imagining acting is subject to the same biomechanical constraints that apply to actual acting.[13]

These same constraints also apply when we observe an action. In the previous chapter we have seen that the rapid sequence of two images, such as those in Fig. 6.1, induce the perception of apparent movement; if the interval between the two images is not too short and is compatible with the execution of the represented movement, the perceived movement respects the biomechanical constraints and so follows the same, longer trajectory that the observer would have used had they been executing the movement themselves. If, on the other hand, the interval between the two images is very short, to the point of not being compatible with the execution of the represented movement, the perceived movement follows the shorter trajectory, even if it constitutes a violation of the biomechanical constraints. These differences will not be present if the two images represent parts of an object (such as the hands of a

---

[13]   As Gregory Currie and Ian Ravenscroft have opportunely pointed out, 'If imagined movement is constrained by the factors which constrain our real movement, it follows that imagining impossible movements is itself impossible. Objecting to this, some people claim to be able to imagine-in a kinesthetically vivid way-such impossible movements as extending their arms so as to touch a light fixture in a high ceiling. We reply that one might easily have the sense of being able to imagine doing this while in fact not being able to. For one thing, kinesthetic imagery is sometimes difficult to distinguish from visual imagery, and there is, on our view, no objection to imagining seeing an arm being thus extended. But more importantly, we grant that it is possible to imagine in a kinesthetic way parts of the process of extending one's arm to the ceiling: you imagine stretching upwards, straining to reach the ceiling; you then imagine actually touching it. Neither of these is biomechanically impossible, but taken together they do not amount, strictly speaking, to imagining stretching to the ceiling. We are prone to describe partial imaginings in terms strictly applicable to the whole: people who imagine swimming 100 yards rarely undertake the whole episode in imagination. It may therefore be that we take a sequence of possible, partial imaginings to be the completion of an act of imagining which, taken as a whole, is actually impossible' (Currie & Ravenscroft, 1997, p. 170).

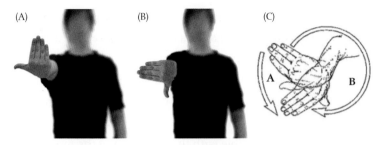

Fig. 6.1 A hand shown in two different positions. If shown in rapid sequence, these two images appear to move clockwise or anti-clockwise in relation to the person's body. In the photo on the left (A), the trajectory is longer, but biomechanically compatible; in the photo on the right (B) it is shorter, but violates biomechanical constraints. In (C) are illustrated the two direction of the perceived hand rotations.

clock). In this case, whatever the duration of the interval, the perceived movement always follows the shorter trajectory.

It is interesting to note that if the observer has a deficit in representing the observed action motorically, it is possible that they will only see the action *from the outside*, representing it in terms of purely visual images with no motor constraints, which is what happens when we observe inanimate objects that move in a mechanical manner (Funk et al., 2005; see also Fiori et al., 2013). If, when we observe a given action, we recruit the same motor processes and representations that would be recruited if we ourselves were to execute that action, the representation will not be very different to that which would be obtained if we were to imagine executing it—and the cerebral areas activated, particularly the parieto-frontal areas, are very similar.[14] For that matter, the capability of imagining executing an action, like the capability of mirroring

[14] See Jeannerod (2001) for an analysis of the similarities and the differences between motor imagination and observation of action. See also Cattaneo et al. (2009).

observed actions, depends on the motor repertoire of the imaginer or the observer: the more expert a person is in executing a given action, the better they will be able to represent it motorically, both when imagining executing it themselves and when observing it being executed by others. In both these cases, the represented action is motorically not so very different from the executed action, except of course for the muscles and tendons involved in the physically executed action.[15]

This representing *from the inside* distinguishes the understanding made possible by the mirror responses and their corresponding sensorimotor transformations. Marc Jeannerod, to whom we owe some of the most brilliant and original analyses of the nature and reach of motor imagery, had already intuited this. In his 2004 paper, *Actions from Within*, he wrote:

> A mere visual perception, without involvement of the motor system, would only provide a description of the visible aspects of the movements of the agent; but it would not give precise information about the intrinsic components of the observed action which are critical for understanding what the action is about, what is its goal, and how to reproduce it. (Jeannerod, 2004, p. 391)

This explains why we are faster and much more accurate in understanding the actions we are observing if we are able to call on the representations and processes induced by mirror responses and their corresponding sensorimotor transformations; also because

---

[15] 'One might even tentatively propose that a covert action includes everything that is involved in an overt action, except for the muscular contractions and the joint rotations. Even though this contention is factually incorrect, as we know that the muscle-articular events associated with a real movement generate a flow of reafferent signals which are not present as such in a covert action, it captures many aspects of the functioning of the representation' (Jeannerod, 2004, p. 379).

we can call on precise information regarding the 'intrinsic components of the observed action': we are not restricted to the external image that can guarantee a purely sensory perception, but we can actually *go inside* the observed action, with the aid of the representations and processes that we would recruit if we were to execute the action ourselves. In other words, all things considered, if when we are observing an action we can call on the representations and processes induced by mirror responses, we will be able to understand it *earlier* and *much better*, because we understand it in a *very different way* compared to how we would understand it on the basis of purely sensory representations and processes.

The concept of understanding *from the inside* is not applicable exclusively to the action domain but extends naturally to the domains of emotion and of vitality forms. In Chapter 3 we saw that while we are observing other people's emotional expressions, we recruit visceromotor processes and representations similar to those we would have recruited if we had imagined experiencing them ourselves—and in both cases the representations and processes involved are similar to those that would be recruited if the emotions were to be actually experienced (see, for example, Jabbi et al., 2007). In addition to this, we can distinguish between representing *from the inside* and representing *from the outside* for emotions. This point is best illustrated by the cases of N.K., B., and S.M., the patients mentioned earlier in this chapter. None of them had significant deficits in their capability of *visually* recognizing facial features, nor did they have difficulty in using concepts or understanding the significance of terms linked to emotions such as disgust or fear. However, none of them could access precise information regarding the 'intrinsic components' of the observed emotional expression—information that would have enabled them to understand which kind of emotion was linked to the facial and bodily expressions they were observing in the other person, the kind of experience involved and the appropriate response to those expressions.

Lastly, what we have seen above applied to actions and emotions appears to be equally valid for vitality forms. We know that in this case too, while we are observing actions executed with a vitality form, the mirror responses recruit motor representations and processes that are not unlike those recruited when we imagine executing those self-same actions with those vitality forms ourselves – and both these cases, in their turn, are similar to those recruited when those actions are physically executed with those vitality forms (see, for example, Di Cesare et al., 2015). Although research in this domain is still in the early stages, it is plausible to assume that, as for actions and emotions, the representations and processes evoked by mirror responses and their corresponding sensorimotor transformations will assist in capturing those 'intrinsic components' of an action that are 'critical' in understanding not only *what*, i.e. the action goal, but also *how*, i.e. the form that identifies the manner in which the action achieves its goal.

The *parallel* between *imagining* acting, feeling an emotion or displaying a vitality form and *observing* other people acting, expressing an emotion or displaying a vitality form provides us with the opportunity to add a *second* characterization to the notion of understanding from the inside. Try to imagine you are moving your fingers over the strings of a guitar in order to play one of Eric Clapton's well-known guitar solos. Unless you are an expert guitarist, it is very unlikely that you will actually be able to do this. However, there is nothing to stop you thinking about playing one of Clapton's solos in the abstract (that is, without imagining actually performing the movements required to play the solo), just as there is nothing to stop you thinking about flying like a bird or a bat, in the abstract. These forms of imagination are mostly *cognitive* in nature and are not bound by the spatial, temporal, and biomechanical constraints that govern motor imagery. As we have seen, motor imagery depends on the capability of representing the action we are imagining motorically; in this it is not unlike the physical execution of the action. All the same, when we say that imagining playing one of Eric Clapton's guitar solos is *almost* like actually playing it, we are not only alluding to the fact that in both cases the *motor processes* and *representations* are *similar*. It is also often suggested that the two *experiences*, the one imagining playing the guitar solo and the other, physically playing it on a real guitar, are surprisingly *similar* at least in part.[16] In this respect, motor imagery differs radically from cognitive imagination: you can think about flying like a bird or a bat, even if you have no idea of what it is like to fly like a bird or a bat.

This last point is crucial because it can be applied, obviously within certain limits, to observing and understanding action. When describing the role of mirror responses and the corresponding sensorimotor transformations, we have frequently underlined how observing an action can evoke processes and representations that are similar to those that would be evoked if the observer were to execute the action themselves. We have also pointed out that in this regard, observing an action is not so very

[16] On this point, see, for example, Currie and Ravenscroft (1997, p. 161) but also Jeannerod and Decety (1995, p. 727), and Kosslyn et al. (2001, pp. 638–639). The same is also applicable to visual imagery; see Gendler (2011), for example.

different from imagining executing that action. However, since *imagining* executing an action—imagining in the sense of motor imagery—can be similar in certain ways to *executing* that action not only from the *representational*, but also from the *phenomenological* point of view, it appears plausible to conclude that the *observation* of an action, when it triggers a mirror response, can be similar in certain ways to the *execution* of the action, not only from the *representational* but also from the *phenomenological* point of view for the observer. In both cases, in fact, our experience of an action, whether we imagine executing it ourselves or whether we see it being executed by others, depends at least partially on how the action is motorically represented. Which is exactly what happens when the action is executed physically.[17]

Think of how your experience executing a certain action varies as your motor expertise in that action increases. And think of how a change in your motor expertise affects your experience in imagining executing that action. The fact that executing an action and imagining it are phenomenologically similar is mainly because both experiences are, in a manner of speaking, *shaped* by motor processes and representations; as your capability of motorically representing an action goal increases—let's say your capability of playing a guitar solo like Clapton, to continue with our previous example—your experience of that action will become richer and

---

[17] To avoid any confusion, it must be pointed out that when we hypothesize a phenomenological resemblance between the experience of executing a given action and that of observing someone else executing an action of that type, we are not referring to that component of the experience of the action known as agency and by which you experience the action as yours rather than mine, but to that which is experienced when an action is executed aimed at one particular goal such as grasping rather throwing or kicking. On this point, see Sinigaglia and Butterfill (2019).

more articulate, whether you are playing a real guitar or just imagining it. Now, imagine observing someone else playing that guitar. Leaving aside the actual sound, your experience in watching the person's fingers moving over the strings will differ according to your own level of expertise in playing the guitar. Once again, the better you are at playing that solo piece, the richer will be your experience when you watch it being played by others. As your mastery of the instrument increases, you will be able to perceive every detail and anticipate possible developments, *almost* as if you yourself were playing the piece.

If, as we believe, the parallel between motor imagery and action observation holds true, it will follow that understanding *from the inside*, enabled by the mirror responses and their corresponding transformations, evokes a resemblance which extends beyond representations and processes to the kind of experience involved. Just as the experience of imagining executing an action can be surprisingly similar to the experience of actually executing it, so the experience of observing an action can, for the observer, be surprisingly similar to the experience they would have were they not merely observing but actually executing it.

This resemblance may be even stronger when we move from the action domain to that of the emotions. Imagine for a moment the disgust you feel at the sight of putrefying food, or the gripping fear you would feel if someone were to threaten you with a knife. Don't limit yourself to just thinking about the possibility of feeling this or that emotion; try to imagine really experiencing it. You will find that, to a certain extent, the experience will not be so very different to that of finding yourself seated in front of that plate of putrefying food or facing a stranger with a knife in a dark alley. In both cases your experience is shaped by visceromotor processes and representations; and it is due to these representations and processes that you can experience these emotions, whether you are actually living them or only imagining them.

Now, imagine that suddenly, out of the blue, you see someone, anyone, reacting in disgust or fear. You may be totally unaware of what provoked this reaction, but the mere sight of that contorted face or recoiling posture will evoke visceromotor processes and representations similar to those that you would recruit were you to experience those emotions yourself. And that is not all; those processes and representations can shape your experience of observing someone else expressing a given emotion in the same way as they shape your own experience of the same emotion. In both cases, your experience depends, at least in part, on the same kind of processes and representations. Indeed, as happened with the imagination, when you observe other people expressing an emotion, your experience will not be unlike your experience of living that emotion yourself.

Emotional contagion is an extreme case of this. You will certainly have experienced a frisson of fear at the sight of a frightened face, or felt a sense of hilarity, even momentarily, on hearing someone enjoying a full-bellied laugh. It is not so surprising that your experience and that of the other person have similar traits in situations such as these. What is surprising, however, is that this holds true – within certain limits – also when observing other people experiencing emotion does not reveal any form of explicit contagion. We know that however much emotional contagion presupposes the capability of mirroring other people's emotions, mirror responses themselves do not imply any form of contagion. However, they do imply a recruitment of those representations and processes that would be recruited if the observer were experiencing the emotion themselves. These representations and processes can shape the observer's experience, rendering it different to the mere visual experience of this or that facial feature, or the posture of this or that body part.

Indeed, this is the experience that appears to be lacking in patients with lesions of the cerebral structures involved in the visceromotor processing and representation of emotions such as fear and disgust. In the preceding pages we have frequently mentioned how patients N.K., B., and S.M. lacked the experience of these emotions and were incapable of understanding them when they encountered them in other people. Not only were they not able to *represent* such emotions visceromotorically, their own *experience* of these emotions was also negatively affected, when it was supposed they would be experiencing them personally. In addition, at least according to the accounts given by these patients, this inability also affected their experience when they observed certain emotional expressions and reactions in other people. You will remember that they did not have any difficulty in conceiving of this or that emotion, nor in understanding, from a conceptual point of view, which reactions would be the most appropriate. Nor did they have any specific sensory or auditive deficits, so their visual and auditive experience was no different to yours. But in spite of this, if we are to rely on their account, what they experienced while observing other people's emotional expressions and reactions was different to what we would experience. That being the case, this difference would seem to depend on the fact that their experience could not be shaped by the visceromotor representations and processes that shape ours. This prevented them from giving 'colour', so to speak, to concepts such as fear and disgust, even though they know the meaning in an abstract sense, and from understanding those emotions from the inside, whether experiencing them themselves or observing others experiencing them.

The Chapter in Brief

Our aim in this chapter was to clarify how mirror responses and their corresponding transformations can play a distinctive role in understanding other people's actions, emotions, and vitality forms.

As an initial step, we explained the distinction between *basic* and *full-blown understanding*; while all that is needed to have a *basic understanding* of an observed action is the capability of representing one or more goals and to realize that the action in question is directed at them, *full-blown understanding* requires, among other things, certain knowledge of the states that can be supposed to have supplied the person carrying out the action with motivating reasons. This is true also for emotions and vitality forms: for example, if all that is needed for a basic understanding of someone else's emotion is the capability of identifying the kind of emotion they are experiencing, a full-blown understanding requires, once more among other things, the capability of explaining why that person, with that character, state of mind, sensibility, and beliefs, was able to experience that kind of emotion in that particular situation.

Making these distinctions was the first step towards clarifying our thesis that mirror neurons and their corresponding transformations play a specific role in understanding other people's actions, emotions, and vitality forms. Analysing the results we have reviewed and discussed in the preceding chapters shows how mirror responses are sufficient in themselves, other things being equal, for a basic understanding of actions, emotions, and vitality forms of other individuals, while at the same time exerting a content-respecting influence on the observer's capability of *judging* them. This has given us the opportunity to respond to some of the objections that have been raised against our claim over the years. In our defence we have argued that the attribution of a specific role to mirror responses in understanding other people's actions and emotions in no way implies that these responses are a necessary condition for understanding the actions and emotions in other people, nor does it imply that any motor or visceromotor deficit will necessarily result in a deficit in understanding actions and emotions. Our claim is in fact perfectly consistent with the possibility that the observer might understand other people's actions and emotions using representations other than those evoked by mirror neurons and their corresponding transformations. In addition, the contrast between mirror-based and non-mirror-based understanding helps to clarify the distinctive role of the mirror responses in understanding action and emotion and their corresponding sensorimotor and visceromotor transformations.

With a view to highlighting what mirror responses have caused to be distinctive to the understanding of actions, emotions, and vitality forms, we have adopted the notion *understanding from the inside*, identifying two different but complementary characterizations of the term. In the first characterization, the term indicates that this kind of understanding depends on the same kind of motor and visceromotor processes and representations that concern the 'intrinsic components' of the actions and the emotions when they are executed or experienced personally rather than being observed while others execute or experience them. This explains why we understand other people's actions and emotions *more accurately* and *much earlier* when we can call on representations induced by mirror responses, as these representations allow us to understand other people's actions and emotions differently to how they would be understood on the basis of inferential processes involving sensory representations.

The second characterization of the term *understanding from the inside* further clarifies how this kind of understanding *differs* from others, regardless of whether or not they have a sensory base. In this second aspect, understanding from the inside is characterized not only by the recruitment of the motor or visceromotor representations that are usually involved in executing an action or feeling an emotion, but rather, and above all, by the fact that these representations can *shape* the experience of an action or an emotion of a certain kind, not only when executing it or feeling it personally, but also when observing someone else executing it or experiencing it. The proof of this lies in the fact that when there is a change in the way an action or an emotion is motorically or visceromotorically represented, our experience of that action or emotion changes also; this is true both when the experience is our own and when we observe it in others. Understanding other people's actions and emotions from the inside presupposes an experience of these actions and emotions which, while obviously different from the experience that underlies executing an action or experiencing an emotion personally, still shares some fundamental aspects with it. To sum up, leaving aside the obvious differences, what you experience when you see someone executing an action or feeling an emotion is similar to what you would experience were you to execute that action or feel that emotion yourself.

CONCLUSION

We have now reached the conclusion of this book. One of our aims was to provide evidence that the mirror property characterizes not only a significant portion of our primate brain, but also of several brain structures of other species which are distant from each other in evolutionary terms. Today, much of the discussion regarding the mirror property and its possible functions still revolves around the data obtained from the parieto-frontal areas involved in the representation of actions. This can probably be attributed to the fact that the first neurons with the mirror property were discovered in the ventral premotor cortex of the brain of the macaque, and the richest and most detailed descriptions of the functional characteristics of mirror neurons currently available are relative to the premotor and parietal areas. Now, however, as we have explained throughout this book, the time has come to correct what today appears to be a classic 'error of prospective' and to acknowledge that not only do many areas possess the mirror property—such as the insula, the amygdala, the cingulate cortex, the hippocampus—but a good number of these are also more ancient from an evolutionary standpoint and functionally more basic than those of the parieto-frontal network.

Mirroring Brains. Giacomo Rizzolatti and Corrado Sinigaglia, Oxford University Press. © Oxford University Press 2023. DOI: 10.1093/oso/9780198871705.003.0007

As long as the mirror property continued to be considered a prerogative of a small portion of the premotor cortex, it was plausible that neurons possessing this property should be thought of on a par with other types of neurons, such as the *place cells* or those that respond selectively to faces. This can no longer be the case, as it is clear that this particular property, the mirror property, involves a wide variety of neurons with different functional characteristics, to the extent that, as we have seen, even place cells can have it. The fundamental difference between the functional characteristics that identify the various types of neurons and the mirror property is that the latter concerns the possibility for the neurons themselves to use their functional characteristics to represent something (e.g. action goals, emotions, vitality forms, and so on) that pertains to itself or to others.

One interesting question is why the mirror property is present in different cerebral areas and in different species. A possible answer to this could be that, at least from an evolutionary standpoint, it is parsimonious and effective to recruit the same neuronal resources for processes and representations that concern oneself and others. In addition, these resources are extremely robust as many are active from the first months of life. Consider the domains that we have covered in the preceding chapters: mirror responses exploit the robustness of the neuronal circuits typically involved in the motor and visceromotor representations underlying most of our daily actions and emotions to process information concerning these when we see them being executed or experienced by other people. It is reasonable to assume that the same happens in the case of other neuronal and representational resources in other species.

Another aim we set ourselves was to clarify if and to what extent mirror responses and their corresponding sensorimotor or sensori-visceromotor transformations play a distinctive role in understanding other people's actions, emotions, and vitality forms. As mentioned, this is one of the most debated questions, if not *the* most debated, of recent years. In Chapters 5 and 6 we have attempted to provide sound reasons, sourcing from experimental and theoretical standpoints, to support the claim that mirror responses are *sufficient*, other things being equal, for a *basic understanding* of the actions, emotions, and vitality forms executed, experienced, and displayed by others, contemporaneously influencing the ability of the observer to *judge* them.

We further characterized this type of understanding, proposing that it be known as *understanding from the inside*, identifying two different but complementary characterizations of the term. The first refers to the fact the mirror responses and their corresponding transformations allow us to *go inside*, in a manner of speaking to penetrate, the actions, emotional reactions, and vitality forms of other people, as we can call into play processes and representations that are similar to those which make possible it possible to execute these same actions, experience emotional reactions, and display vitality forms ourselves. The second regards the possibility that these processes and representations shape our experience of certain kinds of action, emotions, and vitality forms, not only when we ourselves execute, experience, or display them but also when we see them being executed, experienced, or displayed by others. Apart from the obvious differences, executing an action, experiencing an emotion, exhibiting a vitality form ourselves and watching someone doing the same may be phenomenologically similar compared to the action, emotion, or vitality form in question. In short, what we experience while watching someone executing an action or experiencing an emotion is similar, at least in part, to what we ourselves experience when executing that action or feeling that emotion.

This would explain why mirror responses and their corresponding transformations place us in a position to understand what other people are doing or feeling more quickly and accurately than people who do not have access to the same resources in terms of processes, representations, and experiences. This assumes even greater importance if we consider that, as we have frequently pointed out, mirror responses and their corresponding transformations are relative to processes, representations, and experiences that significantly contribute to our ability to successfully interact with other people.

While it is certainly not our place to judge whether we have achieved our aims, we hope that the material we have presented and reviewed in this book will contribute to a better understanding of the mirror mechanism and its potential implications from the experimental and theoretical standpoints. Many challenges await us in the coming years, one of which is to systematically investigate whether the processes fundamental from an evolutionary point of view for the various species are characterized by the mirror property and if so, to what extent. Another challenge is to conduct more detailed studies in primates (but not only) regarding the contributions of the various neuron populations that possess the mirror property to the representations of our own behaviour and that of others. Last, but not least, there is a challenge of particular interest from both the experimental and the theoretical standpoints, that consists in the possibility of integrating in humans the basic understanding that mirror responses can establish with the full-blown understanding frequently attributed to networks that are apparently without the mirror property. As we mentioned earlier, this challenge will require the definition of innovative paradigmatic tasks able to measure the roles and contributions of the various networks, and how these can influence each other; but maybe the most important aspect of this challenge for the future is the need to dedicate an ever increasing degree of attention to the emotional and affective components that play such an important part in our ability to interact with others.

BIBLIOGRAPHY

Abdollahi, R.O., Jastorff, J., Orban, G.A. (2013), 'Common and segregated processing of observed actions in human SPL'. *Cerebral Cortex*, 23, pp. 2734–2753.

Abernethy, B. (2008), 'Motor learning and control activation of the brain's mirror network in anticipatory tasks'. *Journal of Sport Exercise Psychology*, 30, pp. 61–144.

Ackroyd, K., Riddoch, M.J., Humphreys, G.W., Nightingale, S., Townsend, S. (2002), 'Widening the sphere of influence: Using a tool to extend extrapersonal visual space in a patient with severe neglect'. *Neurocase*, 8, pp. 1–12.

Adolphs, R. (2016), 'Human lesion studies in the 21st century'. *Neuron*, 90, pp. 1151–1153.

Adolphs, R., Tranel, D., Damasio, H., Damasio, A.R. (1994), 'Impaired recognition of emotion in facial expressions following bilateral damage to the human amygdala'. *Nature*, 372, pp. 669–672.

Adolphs, R., Tranel, D., Damasio, H., Damasio, A.R. (1995), 'Fear and the human amygdala'. *Journal of Neuroscience*, 15, pp. 5879–5892.

Adolphs, R., Tranel, D., Hamann, S., Young, A.W., Calder, A.J., Phelps, E.A., Lee, G.P., Damasio, A.R. (1999), 'Recognition of facial emotion in nine subjects with bilateral amygdala damage'. *Neuropsychologia*, 37, pp. 1111–1117.

Adolphs, R., Tranel, D., Damasio, A.R. (2003), ' "Dissociable neural systems for recognizing emotions" '. *In Brain Cognition*, 52, pp. 61-–69.

Aglioti, S.M., Cesari, P., Romani, M., Urgesi, C. (2008), 'Action anticipation and motor resonance in elite basketball players'. *Nature Neuroscience*, 11, pp. 1109–1116.

Agnew, Z., Wise, R.J.S. (2008), 'Separate areas for mirror responses and agency within the parietal operculum'. *Journal of Neuroscience*, 28, 47, pp. 12268–12273.

Allen, C. (2010), 'Mirror, mirror in the brain, what's the monkey stand to gain?'. *Noûs*, 44, pp. 372–391.

Almashaikhi, T., Rheims, S., Jung, J., Ostrowsky-Coste, K., Montavont, A., De Bellescize, J., Ryvlin, P. (2014), 'Functional connectivity of insular efferences'. *Human Brain Mapping*, 35, 10, pp. 5279–5294.

Altschuler, E.L., Vankov, A., Wang, V., Ramachandran, V.S., Pineda, J.A. (1997), 'Person see, person do: Human cortical electrophysiological correlates of monkey see monkey do cell'. *Society of Neuroscience Abstracts*, 719, p. 17.

Altschuler, E.L., Vankov, A., Hubbard, E.M., Roberts, E., Ramachandran, V.S., Pineda, J.A. (2000), 'Mu wave blocking by observation of movement and its possible use as a tool to study theory of other minds'. *Society of Neuroscience Abstracts*, 68, p. 1.

Amaral, D.G., Price, J.L. (1984), 'Amygdalo-cortical projections in the monkey (*Macaca fascicularis*)'. *Journal of Comparative Neurology*, 230, 4, pp. 465–496.

Amaral, D.G., Adolphs, R. (2016) (editors), *Living Without an Amygdala*. Guilford Press, New York/London.

Ambrosini, E., Costantini, M., Sinigaglia, C. (2011), 'Grasping with the eyes'. *Journal of Neurophysiology*, 106, 3, pp. 1437–1442.

Ambrosini, E., Sinigaglia, C., Costantini, M. (2012), 'Tie my hands, tie my eyes'. *Journal of Experimental Psychology: Human Perception and Performance*, 38, 2, pp. 263–266.

Ambrosini, E., Reddy, V., De Looper, A., Costantini, M., Lopez, B., Sinigaglia, C. (2013), 'Looking ahead: Anticipatory gaze and motor ability in infancy'. *PLoS One*, 8, 7, e67916.

An, X., Badler, R., Öngür, D., Price, J.L. (1998), 'Prefrontal cortical projections to longitudinal columns in the midbrain periaqueductal gray in macaque monkeys'. *Journal of Comparative Neurology*, 401, 4, pp. 455–479.

Andersen, R.A. (1987), 'Inferior parietal lobule function in spatial perception and visuomotor integration'. In *Handbook of Physiology. The Nervous System. Higher Function of the Brain*, Section 1, Volume 5, Brookhart, J.M., Mountcastle, V.B. (editors). American Physiological Society, Bethesda (MD), pp. 483–518.

Andersen, R.A., Snyder, A.L., Bradley, D.C., Xing, J. (1997), 'Multimodal representation of space in the posterior parietal cortex and its use in planning movements'. *Annual Review of Neuroscience*, 20, pp. 303–330.

Anderson, W., Jaffe, J. (1972), 'The definition, detection and timing of vocalic syllables in speech signals'. *New York State Psychiatric Institute Scientific Report*, 12.

Arbib, M.A., Iberall, T., Lyons, D. (1985), 'Coordinated control programs for control of the hands'. In *Hand Function and the Neocortex, Experimental Brain Research Supplemental*, 10, Goodwin, A.W., Darian-Smith, I. (editors), Springer, Berlin, pp. 14243–14249.

Armony, J., Vuilleumier, P. (2013) (editors), *The Cambridge Handbook of Human Affective Neuroscience*. Cambridge University Press, Cambridge, UK.

Arnstein, D., Cui, F., Keysers, C., Maurits, N.M., Gazzola, V. (2011), 'μ-suppression during action observation and execution correlates with Bold in dorsal premotor, inferior parietal, and SI cortices'. *Journal of Neuroscience*, 31, 40, pp. 14243–14249.

Arroyo, S., Lesser, R.P., Gordon, B., Uematsu, S., Hart, J., Schwerdt, P., Andreasson, K., Fisher, R.S. (1993), 'Mirth, laughter and gelastic seizures'. *Brain*, 116, 4, pp. 757–780.

Bach, D.R., Hurlemann, R., Dolan, R.J. (2015), 'Impaired threat prioritisation after selective bilateral amygdala lesions'. *Cortex*, 63, pp. 206–213.

Bakker, M., Sommerville, J.A., Gredebäck, G. (2016), 'Enhanced neural processing of goal-directed actions after active training in 4-month-old infants'. *Journal of Cognitive Neuroscience*, 28, 3, pp. 472–482.

Bardi, L., Six, P., Brass, M. (2017), 'Repetitive TMS of the temporo-parietal junction disrupts participant's expectations in a spontaneous Theory of Mind task'. *Social Cognitive and Affective Neuroscience*, 12, 11, pp. 1775–1782.

Baumgärtner, U., Tiede, W., Treede, R.D., Craig, A.D. (2006), 'Laser-evoked potentials are graded and somatotopically organized anteroposteriorly in the operculoinsular cortex of anesthetized monkeys'. *Journal of Neurophysiology*, 96, 5, pp. 2802–2808.

Bechara, A., Tranel, D., Damasio, H., Adolphs, R., Rockland, C., Damasio, A.R. (1995), 'Double dissociation of conditioning and declarative knowledge relative to the amygdala and hippocampus in humans'. *Science*, 269, 5227, pp. 1115–1118.

Becker, B., Mihov, Y., Scheele, D., Kendrick, K.M., Feinstein, J.S., Matusch, A., Aydin, M., Reich, H., Urbach, H., Oros-Peusquens, A.M., Shah, N.J., Kunz, W.S., Schlaepfer, T.E., Zilles, K., Maier, W., Hurlemann, R. (2011), 'Fear processing and social networking in the absence of a functional amygdala'. *Biological Psychiatry*, 72, 1, pp. 70–77.

Beets, I.A.M., Rösler, F., Fiehler, K. (2010), 'Nonvisual motor learning improves visual motion perception: Evidence from violating the two-thirds power law'. *Journal of Neurophysiology*, 104, 3, pp. 1612–1624.

Belmalih, A., Borra, E., Contini, M., Gerbella, M., Rozzi, S., Luppino, G. (2007), 'A multiarchitectonic approach for the definition of functionally distinct areas and domains in the monkey frontal lobe'. *Journal of Anatomy*, 211, pp. 199–211.

Belmalih, A., Borra, E., Contini, M., Gerbella, M., Rozzi, S., Luppino, G. (2009), 'Multimodal architectonic subdivision of the rostral part (area F5) of the macaque ventral premotor cortex'. *Journal of Comparative Neurology*, 512, 2, pp. 183–217.

Bernstein, M., Yovel, G. (2015), 'Two neural pathways of face processing: A critical evaluation of current models'. *Neuroscience and Biobehavioral Reviews*, 55, pp. 536–546.

Berti, A., Frassinetti, F. (2000), 'When far becomes near: Re-mapping of space by tool use'. *Journal of Cognitive Neuroscience*, 12, pp. 415–420.

Berti, A., Smania, N., Rabuffetti, M., Ferrarin, M., Spinazzola, L., D'Amico, A., Ongaro, E., Allport, A. (2002), 'Coding of far and near space during walking in neglect patients'. *Neuropsychology*, 16, 3, pp. 390–399.

Bishop, D.T., Wright, M.J., Jackson, R.C., Abernethy, B. (2013), 'Neural bases for anticipation skill in soccer: An fMRI study'. *Journal of Sport and Exercise Psychology*, 35, 1, pp. 98–109.

Blake, R., Shiffrar, M. (2007), 'Perception of human motion'. *Annual Review of Psychology*, 58, 1, pp. 47–73.

Blakemore, S.J., Bristow, D., Bird, G., Frith, C., Ward, J. (2005), 'Somatosensory activations during the observation of touch and a case of vision-touch synaesthesia'. *Brain*, 128, 7, pp. 1571–1583.

Bonini, L., Rozzi, S., Serventi, F.U., Simone, L., Ferrari, P.F., Fogassi, L. (2010), 'Ventral premotor and inferior parietal cortices make distinct contribution to action organization and intention understanding'. *Cerebral Cortex*, 20, 6, pp. 1372–1385.

Bonini, L., Maranesi, M., Livi, A., Fogassi, L., Rizzolatti, G. (2014), 'Ventral premotor neurons encoding representations of action during self and others' inaction'. *Current Biology*, 24, 14, pp. 1611–1614.

Boria, S., Fabbri-Destro, M., Cattaneo, L., Sparaci, L., Sinigaglia, C., Santelli, E., Cossu, G., Rizzolatti, G. (2009), 'Intention understanding in autism'. *PLoS One*, 4, 5, e5596.

Borra, E., Belmalih, A., Calzavara, R., Gerbella, M., Murata, A., Rozzi, S., Luppino, G. (2008), 'Cortical connections of the macaque anterior intraparietal (AIP) area'. *Cerebral Cortex*, 18, 5, pp. 1094–1111.

Borra, E., Belmalih, A., Gerbella, M., Rozzi, S., Luppino, G. (2010), 'Projections of the hand field of the macaque ventral premotor area F5 to the brainstem and spinal cord'. *Journal of Comparative Neurology*, 518, 13, pp. 2570–2591.

Borra, E., Gerbella, M., Rozzi, S., Luppino, G. (2011), 'Anatomical evidence for the involvement of the macaque ventrolateral prefrontal area 12r in controlling goal-directed actions'. *Journal of Neuroscience*, 31, 34, pp. 12351–12363.

Borra, E., Gerbella, M., Rozzi, S., Luppino, G. (2017), 'The macaque lateral grasping network: A neural substrate for generating purposeful hand actions'. *Neuroscience Biobehavioral Reviews*, 75, pp. 65–90.

Bortoletto, M., Mattingley, J.B., Cunnington, R. (2011), 'Action intentions modulate visual processing during action perception'. *Neuropsychologia*, 49, 7, pp. 2097–2104.

Brass, M., Bekkering, H., Wohlschläger, A., Prinz, W. (2000), 'Compatibility between observed and executed finger movements: Comparing symbolic, spatial, and imitative cues'. *Brain and Cognition*, 44, 2, pp. 124–143.

Brass, M., Bekkering, H., Prinz, W. (2001), 'Movement observation affects movement execution in a simple response task'. *Acta Psychologica*, 106, 1–2, pp. 3–22.

Brass, M., Schmitt, R.M., Spengler, S., Gergely, G. (2007), 'Investigating action understanding: Inferential processes versus action simulation'. *Current Biology*, 17, 24, pp. 2117–2121.

Bråten, S. (1998) (editor), *Intersubjective Communication and Emotion in Early Ontogeny*. Cambridge University Press, Cambridge, UK.

Brodmann, K. (1909), *Vergleichende Lokalisationslehre der Grosshirnrinde in ihren Prinzipien dargestellt auf Grund des Zellenbaues*. Barth, Leipzig.

Broks, P., Young, A.W., Maratos, E.J., Coffey, P.J., Calder, A.J., Isaac, C.L., Mayes, A.R., Hodges, J.R., Montaldi, D., Cezayirli, E., Roberts, N., Hadley, D. (1998), 'Face processing impairments after encephalitis: Amygdala damage and recognition of fear'. *Neuropsychologia*, 36, 1, pp. 59–70.

Bruni, S., Gerbella, M., Bonini, L., Borra, E., Coudé, G., Ferrari, P.F., Fogassi, L., Maranesi, M., Rodà, F., Simone, L., Serventi, F.U., Rozzi, S. (2018), 'Cortical and subcortical connections of parietal and premotor nodes of the monkey hand mirror neuron network'. *Brain Structure and Function*, 223, 4, pp. 1713–1729.

Bub, D.N., Masson, M.E.J. (2010), 'Grasping beer mugs: On the dynamics of alignment effects induced by handled objects'. *Journal of Experimental Psychology: Human Perception and Performance*, 36, 2, pp. 341–358.

Buccino, G., Binkofski, F., Fink, G.R., Fadiga, L., Fogassi, L., Gallese, V., Seitz, R.J., Zilles, K., Rizzolatti, G., Freund, H.-J. (2001), 'Action observation activates premotor and parietal areas in a somatotopic manner: An fMRI study'. *European Journal of Neuroscience*, 13, pp. 400–404.

Buccino, G., Lui, F., Canessa, N., Patteri, I., Lagravinese, G., Benuzzi, F., Porro, C.A., Rizzolatti, G. (2004), 'Neural circuits involved in the recognition of actions performed by non con-specifics: An fMRI study'. *Journal of Cognitive Neuroscience*, 16, pp. 114–126.

Butterfill, S.A., Sinigaglia, C. (2014), 'Intention and motor representation in purposive action'. *Philosophy and Phenomenological Research*, 88, 1, pp. 119–145.

Butterworth, G., Verweij, E., Hopkins, B. (1997), 'The development of prehension in infants: Halverson revisited'. *British Journal of Developmental Psychology*, 15, 2, pp. 223–236.

Buxbaum, L.J., Kyle, K., Grossman, M., Coslett, H.B. (2007), 'Left inferior parietal representations for skilled hand-object interactions: Evidence from stroke and corticobasal degeneration'. *Cortex*, 43, 3, pp. 411–423.

Buxbaum, L.J., Shapiro, A.D., Coslett, H.B. (2014), 'Critical brain regions for tool-related and imitative actions: A componential analysis'. *Brain*, 137, 7, pp. 1971–1985.

Caggiano, V., Fogassi, L., Rizzolatti, G., Thier, P., Casile, A. (2009), 'Mirrror neurons differentially encode the peripersonal and extrapersonal space of monkeys'. *Science*, 324, 5925, pp. 403–406.

Calder, A.J., Keane, J., Manes, F., Antoun, N., Young, A.W. (2000), 'Impaired recognition and experience of disgust following brain injury'. *Nature Neuroscience*, 3, pp. 1077–1078.

Calvo-Merino, B., Glaser, D.E., Grèzes, J., Passingham, R.E., Haggard, P. (2005), 'Action observation and acquired motor skills: An fMRI study with expert dancers'. *Cerebral Cortex*, 15, 8, pp. 1243–1249.

Calvo-Merino, B., Grèzes, J., Glaser, D.E., Passingham, R.E., Haggard, P. (2006), 'Seeing or doing? Influence of visual and motor familiarity in action observation'. *Current Biology*, 16, 19, pp. 1905–1910.

Candidi, M., Urgesi, C., Ionta, S., Aglioti, S.M. (2008), 'Virtual lesion of ventral premotor cortex impairs visual perception of biomechanically possible but not impossible actions'. *Social Neuroscience*, 3, 3–4, pp. 388–400.

Candidi, M., Sacheli, L.M., Mega, I., Aglioti, S.M. (2014), 'Somatotopic mapping of piano fingering errors in sensorimotor experts: TMS studies in pianists and visually trained musically naïves'. *Cerebral Cortex*, 24, 2, pp. 435–443.

Canessa, N., Motterlini, M., Di Dio, C., Perani, D., Scifo, P., Cappa, S.F., Rizzolatti, G. (2009), 'Understanding others' regret: A fMRI study'. *PLoS One*, 4, 10, e7402.

Cannon, E.N., Woodward, A.L. (2012), 'Infants generate goal-based action predictions'. *Developmental Science*, 15, 2, pp. 292–298.

Caramazza, A., Anzellotti, S., Strnad, L., Lingnau, A. (2014), 'Embodied cognition and mirror neurons: A critical assessment'. *Annual Review of Neuroscience*, 37, 1, pp. 1–15.

Cardellicchio, P., Sinigaglia, C., Costantini, M. (2011), 'The space of affordances: A TMS study'. *Neuropsychologia*, 49, 5, pp. 1369–1372.

Cardellicchio, P., Sinigaglia, C., Costantini, M. (2013), 'Grasping affordances with the other's hand: A TMS study'. *Social Cognitive and Affective Neuroscience*, 8, 4, pp. 455–459.

Carmichael, S.T., Price, J.L. (1995), 'Sensory and premotor connections of the orbital and medial prefrontal cortex of macaque monkeys'. *Journal of Comparative Neurology*, 363, 4, pp. 642–664.

Carr, L., Iacoboni, M., Dubeau, M.C., Mazziotta, J.C., Lenzi, G.L. (2003), 'Neural mechanisms of empathy in humans'. *Proceedings of the National Academy of Sciences of the United States of America*, 100, 9, pp. 5497–5502.

Caruana, F., Jezzini, A., Sbriscia-Fioretti, B., Rizzolatti, G., Gallese, V. (2011), 'Emotional and social behaviors elicited by electrical stimulation of the Insula in the macaque monkey'. *Current Biology*, 21, 3, pp. 195–199.

Caruana, F., Avanzini, P., Gozzo, F., Francione, S., Cardinale, F., Rizzolatti, G. (2015), 'Mirth and laughter elicited by electrical stimulation of the human anterior cingulate cortex'. *Cortex*, 71, pp. 323–331.

Caruana, F., Avanzini, P., Gozzo, F., Pelliccia, V., Casaceli, G., Rizzolatti, G. (2017), 'A mirror mechanism for smiling in the anterior cingulate cortex'. *Emotion*, 17, 2, pp. 187–190.

Caruana, F., Gerbella, M., Avanzini, P., Gozzo, F., Pelliccia, V., Mai, R., Abdollahi, R.O., Cardinale, F., Sartori, I., Lo Russo, G., Rizzolatti, G. (2018), 'Motor and emotional behaviours elicited by electrical stimulation of the human cingulate cortex'. *Brain*, 141, 10, pp. 3035–3051.

Casartelli, L., Cesareo, A., Biffi, E., Campione, G.C., Villa, L., Molteni, M., Sinigaglia, C. (2020), 'Vitality form expression in autism'. *Scientific Reports*, 10, 17182.

Casartelli, L., Federici, A., Fumagalli, L., Cesareo, A., Nicoli, M., Ronconi, L., Vitale, A., Molteni, M., Rizzolatti, G., Sinigaglia, C. (2020), 'Neurotypical individuals fail to understand action vitality form in children with autism spectrum disorder.' *Proceedings of the National Academy of Sciences of the United States of America*, 117, pp. 27712–27718.

Casile, A., Giese, M.A. (2006), 'Nonvisual motor training influences biological motion perception'. *Current Biology*, 16, 1, pp. 69–74.

Caspers, S., Zilles, K., Laird, A.R., Eickhoff, S.B. (2010), 'ALE meta-analysis of action observation and imitation in the human brain'. *NeuroImage*, 50, 3, pp. 1148–1167.

Catenoix, H., Isnard, J., Guénot, M., Petit, J., Remy, C., Mauguière, F. (2008), 'The role of the anterior insular cortex in ictal vomiting: A stereotactic electroencephalography study'. *Epilepsy Behavior*, 13, pp. 560–563.

Cattaneo, L., Fabbri-Destro, M., Boria, S., Pieraccini, C., Monti, A., Cossu, G., Rizzolatti, G. (2007), 'Impairment of actions chains in autism and its possible role in intention understanding'. *Proceedings of the National Academy of Sciences*, 104, 45, pp. 17825–17830.

Cattaneo, L., Caruana, F., Jezzini, A., Rizzolatti, G. (2009), 'Representation of goal and movements without overt motor behavior in the human motor cortex: A transcranial magnetic stimulation study'. *Journal of Neuroscience*, 29, 36, pp. 11134–11138.

Cattaneo, L., Sandrini, M., Schwarzbach, J. (2010), 'State-dependent TMS reveals a hierarchical representation of observed acts in the temporal, parietal, and premotor cortices'. *Cerebral Cortex*, 20, 9, pp. 2252–2258.

Cattaneo, L., Barchiesi, G., Tabarelli, D., Arfeller, C., Sato, M., Glenberg, A.M. (2011), 'One's motor performance predictably modulates the understanding of others' actions through adaptation of premotor visuomotor neurons'. *Social Cognitive and Affective Neuroscience*, 6, 3, pp. 301–310.

Cattaneo, L., Pavesi, G. (2014), 'The facial motor system'. *Neuroscience and Biobehavioral Reviews*, 38, pp. 135–159.

Cipolloni, P.B., Pandya, D.N. (1999), 'Cortical connections of the fronto-parietal opercular areas in the rhesus monkey'. *Journal of Comparative Neurology*, 403, 4, pp. 431–458.

Cisek, P., Kalaska, J.F. (2004), 'Neural correlates of mental rehearsal in dorsal premotor cortex'. *Nature*, 431, 7011, pp. 993–996.

Cochin, S., Barthélémy, B., Roux, S., Martineau, J. (1999), 'Observation and execution of movement: Similarities demonstrated by quantified electroencephalography'. *European Journal of Neuroscience*, 11, pp. 1839–1842.

Colby, C.L., Duhamel, J.-R., Goldberg, M.E. (1993), 'Ventral intraparietal area of the macaque: Anatomic location and visual response properties'. *Journal of Neurophysiology*, 69, 3, pp. 902–914.

Colby, C.L., Goldberg, M.E. (1999), 'Space and attention in parietal cortex'. *Annual Review of Neuroscience*, 22, 1, pp. 319–349.

Cook, R., Bird, G., Catmur, C., Press, C., Heyes, C. (2014), 'Mirror neurons: From origin to function'. *Behavioural and Brain Sciences*, 37, 2, pp. 177–192.

Corbetta, M., Patel, G., Shulman, G.L. (2008), 'The reorienting system of the human brain: From environment to theory of mind'. *Neuron*, 58, 3, pp. 306–324.

Costantini, M., Committeri, G., Galati, G. (2008), 'Effector- and target-independent representation of observed actions: Evidence from incidental repetition priming'. *Experimental Brain Research*, 188, 3, pp. 341–351.

Costantini, M., Ambrosini, E., Tieri, G., Sinigaglia, C., Committeri, G. (2010), 'Where does an object trigger an action? An investigation about affordances in space'. *Experimental Brain Research*, 207, 1–2, pp. 95–103.

Costantini, M., Ambrosini, E., Sinigaglia, C., Gallese, V. (2011), 'Tool-use observation makes far objects ready-to-hand'. *Neuropsychologia*, 49, 9, pp. 2658–63.

Costantini, M., Committeri, G., Sinigaglia, C. (2011), 'Ready both to your and to my hands: Mapping the action space of others'. *PLoS One*, 6, 4, e17923.

Costantini, M., Ambrosini, E., Sinigaglia, C. (2012a), 'Does how I look at what you're doing depend on what I'm doing?'. *Acta Psychologica*, 141, 2, pp. 199–204.

Costantini, M., Ambrosini, E., Sinigaglia, C. (2012b), 'Out of your hand's reach, out of my eyes' reach'. *Quarterly Journal of Experimental Psychology*, 65, 5, pp. 848–855.

Costantini, M., Ambrosini, E., Cardellicchio, P., Sinigaglia, C. (2014), 'How your hand drives my eyes'. *Social Cognitive and Affective Neuroscience*, 9, 5, pp. 705–711.

Costantini, M., Frassinetti, F., Maini, M., Ambrosini, E., Gallese, V., Sinigaglia, C. (2014), 'When a laser pen becomes a stick: remapping of space by tool-use observation in hemispatial neglect'. *Experimental Brain Research*, 232, 10, pp. 3233–3241.

Craig, A.D. (2002), 'How do you feel? Interoception: the sense of the physiological condition of the body'. *Nature Review Neuroscience*, 3, pp. 655–666.

Craig, A.D. (2014), 'Topographically organized projection to posterior insular cortex from the posterior portion of the ventral medial nucleus in the long-tailed macaque monkey'. *Journal of Comparative Neurology*, 522, 1, pp. 36–63.

Craighero, L., Fadiga, L., Rizzolatti, G., Umiltà, C. (1999), 'Action for perception: A motor-visual attentional effect'. *Journal of Experimental Psychology. Human Perception and Performance*, 25, 6, pp. 1673–1692.

Craighero, L., Bello, A., Fadiga, L., Rizzolatti, G. (2002), 'Hand action preparation influences the responses to hand pictures'. *Neuropsychologia*, 40, 5, pp. 492–502.

Cross, E.S., Hamilton, A.F.C., Grafton, S.T. (2006), 'Building a motor simulation de novo: Observation of dance by dancers'. *NeuroImage*, 31, 3, pp. 1257–1267.

Csibra, G. (2007), 'Action mirroring and action interpretation: An alternative account'. In *Sensorimotor Foundations of Higher Cognition. Attention and Performance*, Haggard, P., Rossetti, Y., Kawato, M. (editors), XXII. Oxford University Press, Oxford, pp. 427–451.

Currie, G., Ravenscroft, I. (1997), 'Mental simulation and motor imagery'. *Philosophy of Science*, 64, 1, pp. 161–180.

D'Ausilio, A., Altenmüller, E., Olivetti Belardinelli, M., Lotze, M. (2006), 'Cross-modal plasticity of the motor cortex while listening to a rehearsed musical piece'. *European Journal of Neuroscience*, 24, 3, pp. 955–958.

Damasio, A.R. (1999), *The Feeling of What Happens: Body and Emotion in the Making of Consciousness*. Harcourt Brace, CA.

Danjo, T., Toyoizumi, T., Fujisawa, S. (2018), 'Spatial representations of self and other in the hippocampus'. *Science*, 359, 6372, pp. 213–218.

Darwin, C. (1872), 'The expression of the emotions'. In *Man and Animals*. 1879. John Murray, London.

De Lange, F.P., Spronk, M., Willems, R.M., Toni, I., Bekkering, H. (2008), 'Complementary systems for understanding action intentions'. *Current Biology*, 18, 6, pp. 454–457.

De Renzi, E., Faglioni, P. (1999), 'Apraxia'. In *Handbook of Clinical and Experimental Neuropsychology*, Denes, G., Pizzamiglio, L. (editors). Psychology Press, Hove, pp. 421–440.

De Waal, F.B.M., Preston, S.D. (2017), 'Mammalian empathy: Behavioural manifestations and neural basis'. *Nature Reviews Neuroscience*, 18, 8, pp. 498–509.

Deacon, T.W. (1992), 'Cortical connections of the inferior arcuate sulcus cortex in the macaque brain'. *Brain Research*, 573, 1, pp. 8–26.

Decety, J. (1996), 'Do imagined and executed actions share the same neural substrate?'. *Cognitive Brain Research*, 3, 2, pp. 87–93.

Decety, J., Jeannerod, M., Prablanc, C. (1989), 'The timing of mentally represented actions'. *Behavioural Brain Research*, 34, 1–2, pp. 35–42.

Devinsky, O., Morrell, M.J., Vogt, B.A. (1995), 'Contributions of anterior cingulate cortex to behaviour'. *Brain: A Journal of Neurology*, 118, 1, pp. 279–306.

Di Cesare, G., Di Dio, C., Rochat, M.J., Sinigaglia, C., Bruschweiler-Stern, N., Stern, D.N., Rizzolatti, G. (2014), 'The neural correlates of 'vitality form' recognition: An fMRI study'. *Social Cognitive and Affective Neuroscience*, 9, 7, pp. 951–960.

Di Cesare, G., Di Dio, C., Marchi, M., Rizzolatti, G. (2015), 'Expressing our internal states and understanding those of others'. *Proceedings of the National Academy of Sciences*, 112, 33, pp. 10331–10335.

Di Cesare, G., Fasano, F., Errante, A., Marchi, M., Rizzolatti, G. (2016), 'Understanding the internal states of others by listening to action verbs'. *Neuropsychologia*, 89, pp. 172–179.

Di Cesare, G., Valente, G., Di Dio, C., Ruffaldi, E., Bergamasco, M., Goebel, R., Rizzolatti, G. (2016), 'Vitality forms processing in the insula during action observation: A multivoxel pattern analysis'. *Frontiers in Human Neuroscience*, 10, p. 267.

Di Cesare, G., Marchi, M., Errante, A., Fasano, F., Rizzolatti, G. (2018), 'Mirroring the social aspects of speech and actions: The role of the insula'. *Cerebral Cortex*, 28, 4, pp. 1–10.

Di Cesare, G., Pinardi, C., Carapelli, C., Caruana, F., Marchi, M., Gerbella, M., Rizzolatti, G. (2019), 'Insula connections with the parieto-frontal circuit for generating arm actions in humans and macaque monkeys'. *Cerebral Cortex*, 29, 5, pp. 2140–2147.

Di Dio, C., Di Cesare, G., Higuchi, S., Roberts, N., Vogt, S., Rizzolatti, G. (2013), 'The neural correlates of velocity processing during the observation of a biological effector in the parietal and premotor cortex'. *NeuroImage*, 64, 1, pp. 425–436.

Di Pellegrino, G., Fadiga, L., Fogassi, L., Gallese, V., Rizzolatti, G. (1992), 'Understanding motor events: A neurophysiological study'. *Experimental Brain Research*, 91, pp. 176–180.

Dimberg, U. (1982), 'Facial reactions to facial expressions'. *Psychophysiology*, 19, 6, pp. 643–647.

Dimberg, U. (1990), 'Facial electromyographic reactions and autonomic activity to auditory stimuli'. *Biological Psychology*, 31, pp. 137–147.

Dimberg, U., Thunberg, M. (1998), 'Rapid facial reactions to emotional facial expressions'. *Scandinavian Journal of Psychology*, 39, 1, pp. 39–45.

Dimberg, U., Thunberg, M., Elmehed, K. (2000), 'Unconscious facial reactions to emotional facial expressions'. *Psychological Science*, 11, 1, pp. 86–89.

Dimberg, U., Thunberg, M., Grunedal, S. (2002), 'Facial reactions to emotional stimuli: Automatically controlled emotional responses'. *Cognition and Emotion*, 16, 4, pp. 449–471.

Dolan, R.J., Morris, J.S., De Gelder, B. (2001), 'Crossmodal binding of fear in voice and face'. *Proceedings of the National Academy of Sciences*, 98, 17, pp. 10006–10010.

Downing, P.E., Jiang, Y., Shuman, M., Kanwisher, N. (2001), 'A cortical area selective for visual processing of the human body'. *Science*, 293, 5539, pp. 2470–2473.

Drost, U.C., Rieger, M., Prinz, W. (2007), 'Instrument specificity in experienced musicians'. *Quarterly Journal of Experimental Psychology*, 60, 4, pp. 527–533.

Duhamel, J.-R., Colby, C.L., Goldberg, M.E. (1998), 'Ventral intraparietal area of the macaque: Congruent visual and somatic response properties'. *Journal of Neurophysiology*, 79, 1, pp. 126–136.

Dum, R.P., Strick, P.L. (2005), 'Frontal lobe inputs to the digit representations of the motor areas on the lateral surface of the hemisphere'. *Journal of Neuroscience*, 25, 6, pp. 1375–1386.

Dum, R.P., Levinthal, D.J., Strick, P.L. (2009), 'The spinothalamic system targets motor and sensory areas in the cerebral cortex of monkeys'. *Journal of Neuroscience*, 29, 45, pp. 14223–14235.

Dushanova, J., Donoghue, J. (2010), 'Neurons in primary motor cortex engaged during action observation'. *European Journal of Neuroscience*, 31, pp. 386–398.

Ellis, R., Tucker, M. (2000), 'Micro-affordance: The potentiation of components of action by seen objects'. *British Journal of Psychology*, 91, 4, pp. 451–471.

Fadiga, L., Fogassi, L., Pavesi, G., Rizzolatti, G. (1995), 'Motor facilitation during action observation: A magnetic stimulation study'. *Journal of Neurophysiology*, 73, 6, pp. 2608–2611.

Farnè, A., Làdavas, E. (2000), 'Dynamic size-change of hand peripersonal space following tool use'. *NeuroReport*, 11, 8, pp. 1645–1649.

Farnè, A., Bonifazi, S., Làdavas, E. (2005), 'The role played by tool-use and tool-length on the plastic elongation of peri-hand space: A single case study'. *Cognitive Neuropsychology*, 22, 3–4, pp. 408–418.

Farrow, D., Abernethy, B. (2003), 'Do expertise and the degree of perception-action coupling affect natural anticipatory performance?'. *Perception*, 32, 9, pp. 1127–1139.

Feinstein, J.S., Adolphs, R., Damasio, A., Tranel, D. (2011), 'The human amygdala and the induction and experience of fear'. *Current Biology*, 21, 1, pp. 34–38.

Feinstein, J.S., Buzza, C., Hurlemann, R., Follmer, R.L., Dahdaleh, N.S., Coryell, W.H., Tranel, D., Wemmie, J.A. (2013), 'Fear and panic in humans with bilateral amygdala damage'. *Nature Neuroscience*, 16, 3, pp. 270–272.

Feinstein, J.S., Adolphs, R., Tranel, D. (2016), 'A tale from the world of patient SM'. In *Living Without an Amygdala*, Amaral, D.G., Adolphs, R. (editors). Guilford Press, New York.

Fernández-Baca Vaca, G., Lüders, H.O., Basha, M.M., Miller, J.P. (2011), 'Mirth and laughter elicited during brain stimulation'. *Epileptic Disorders*, 13, pp. 435–440.

Filimon, F., Nelson, J.D., Hagler, D.J., Sereno, M.I. (2007), 'Human cortical representations for reaching: Mirror neurons for execution, observation, and imagery'. *NeuroImage*, 37, 4, pp. 1315–1328.

Finkelstein, A., Derdikman, D., Rubin, A., Foerster, J.N., Las, L., Ulanovsky, N. (2015), 'Three-dimensional head-direction coding in the bat brain'. *Nature*, 517, pp. 159–164.

Fiori, F., Sedda, A., Ferrè, E.R., Toraldo, A., Querzola, M., Pasotti, F., Ovadia, D., Piroddi, C., Dell'Acquila, R., Lunetta, C., Corbo, M., Bottini, G. (2013), 'Exploring motor and visual imagery in amyotrophic lateral sclerosis'. *Experimental Brain Research*, 226, 4, pp. 537–547.

Flanagan, J.R., Johansson, R.S. (2003), 'Action plans used in action observation'. *Nature*, 424, 6950, pp. 769–771.

Flynn, F.G. (1999), 'Anatomy of the insula functional and clinical correlates'. *Aphasiology*, 13, 1, pp. 55–78.

Fogassi, L., Gallese, V., Di Pellegrino, G., Fadiga, L., Gentilucci, M., Luppino, G., Matelli, M., Pedotti, A., Rizzolatti, G. (1992), 'Space coding by premotor cortex'. *Experimental Brain Research*, 89, pp. 686–690.

Fogassi, L., Gallese, V., Fadiga, L., Luppino, G., Matelli, M., Rizzolatti, G. (1996), 'Coding of peripersonal space in inferior premotor cortex (F4)'. *Journal of Neurophysiology*, 76, pp. 141–157.

Fogassi, L., Gallese, V., Buccino, G., Craighero, L., Fadiga, L., Rizzolatti, G. (2001), 'Cortical mechanism for the visual guidance of hand grasping movements in the monkey'. *Brain*, 124, pp. 571–586.

Fogassi, L., Ferrari, P.F., Geslerich, B., Rozzi, S., Chersi, F., Rizzolatti, G. (2005), 'Parietal lobe: From action organisation to intention understanding'. *Science*, 308, pp. 662–667.

Frak, V., Paulignan, Y., Jeannerod, M. (2001), 'Orientation of the opposition axis in mentally simulated grasping'. *Experimental Brain Research*, 136, 1, pp. 120–127.

Fried, I., Wilson, C.L., Macdonald, K.A., Behnke, E.J. (1998), 'Electric current stimulates laughter'. *Nature*, 391, 6668, pp. 650.

Friston, K., Mattout, J., Kilner, J. (2011), 'Action understanding and active inference'. *Biological Cybernetics*, 104, 1–2, pp. 137–160.

Frith, U., Frith, C.D. (2003), 'Development and neurophysiology of mentalizing'. *Philosophical Transactions of the Royal Society B: Biological Sciences*, 358, 1431, pp. 459–473.

Frontera, J.G. (1956), 'Some results obtained by electrical stimulation of the cortex of the island of Reil in the brain of the monkey (*Macaca mulatta*)'. *Journal of Comparative Neurology*, 105, pp. 365–394.

Funk, M., Shiffrar, M., Brugger, P. (2005), 'Hand movement observation by individuals born without hands: Phantom limb experience constrains visual limb perception'. *Experimental Brain Research*, 164, 3, pp. 341–346.

Furl, N., Hadj-Bouziane, F., Liu, N., Averbeck, B.B., Ungerleider, L.G. (2012), 'Dynamic and static facial expressions decoded from motion-sensitive areas in the macaque monkey'. *Journal of Neuroscience*, 32, 45, pp. 15952–15962.

Fusar-Poli, P., Placentino, A., Carletti, F., Landi, P., Allen, P., Surguladze, S., Benedetti, F., Abbamonte, M., Gasparotti, R., Barale, F., Perez, J., McGuire, P., Politi, P. (2009), 'Functional atlas of emotional faces processing: A voxel-based meta-analysis of 105 functional magnetic resonance imaging studies'. *Journal of Psychiatry and Neuroscience*, 34, 6, pp. 418–432.

Gallese, V., Murata, A., Kaseda, M., Niki, N., Sakata, H. (1994), 'Deficit of hand preshaping after mucimol injection in monkey parietal cortex'. *NeuroReport*, 5, pp. 1525–1529.

Gallese, V., Fadiga, L., Fogassi, L., Rizzolatti, G. (1996), 'Action recognition in the premotor cortex'. *Brain*, 119, pp. 593–609.

Gallese, V., Fadiga, L., Fogassi, L., Rizzolatti, G. (2002), 'Action representation and the inferior parietal lobule'. In *Attention and Performance XIX: Common Mechanisms in Perception and Action*, Prinz, W., Hommel, B. (editors). Oxford University Press, Oxford, pp. 247–266.

Gallese, V., Keysers, C., Rizzolatti, G. (2004), 'A unifying view of the basis of social cognition'. *Trends in Cognitive Sciences*, 8, 9, pp. 396–403.

Gallese, V., Sinigaglia, C. (2011), 'What is so special about embodied simulation?'. *Trends in Cognitive Sciences*, 15, 11, pp. 512–519.

Gazzola, V., Aziz-Zadeh, L., Keysers, C. (2006), 'Empathy and the somatotopic auditory mirror system in humans'. *Current Biology*, 16, 18, pp. 1824–1829.

Gazzola, V., Rizzolatti, G., Wicker, B., Keysers, C. (2007), 'The anthropomorphic brain: The mirror neuron system responds to human and robotic actions'. *NeuroImage*, 35, 4, pp. 1674–1684.

Gazzola, V., Van Der Worp, H., Mulder, T., Wicker, B., Rizzolatti, G., Keysers, C. (2007), 'Aplasics born without hands mirror the goal of hand actions with their feet'. *Current Biology*, 17, 14, pp. 1235–1240.

Gazzola, V., Keysers, C. (2009), 'The observation and execution of actions share motor and somatosensory voxels in all tested subjects: Single-subject analyses of unsmoothed fMRI data'. *Cerebral Cortex*, 19, 6, pp. 1239–1255.

Gendler, T. (2011), 'Imagination'. In *The Stanford Encyclopedia of Philosophy*, Zalta, E.N. (editor), Fall 2011 edition. Available at: https://plato.stanford.edu/entries/imagination/

Gentilucci, M., Fogassi, L., Luppino, G., Matelli, M., Camarda, R., Rizzolatti, G. (1988), 'Functional organization of inferior area 6 in the macaque monkey: I. Somatotopy and the control of proximal movements'. *Experimental Brain Research*, 33, 2–3, pp. 118–121.

Gerbella, M., Belmalih, A., Borra, E., Rozzi, S., Luppino, G. (2011), 'Cortical connections of the anterior (F5a) subdivision of the macaque ventral premotor area F5'. *Brain Structure and Function*, 216, 1, pp. 43–65.

Gerbella, M., Borra, E., Tonelli, S., Rozzi, S., Luppino, G. (2013), 'Connectional heterogeneity of the ventral part of the macaque area 46'. *Cerebral Cortex*, 23, 4, pp. 967–987.

Gerbella, M., Baccarini, M., Borra, E., Rozzi, S., Luppino, G. (2014), 'Amygdalar connections of the macaque areas 45A and 45B'. *Brain Structure and Function*, 219, 3, pp. 831–842.

Gerbella, M., Borra, E., Rozzi, S., Luppino, G. (2016), 'Connections of the macaque Granular Frontal Opercular (GrFO) area: A possible neural substrate for the contribution of limbic inputs for controlling hand and face/mouth actions'. *Brain Structure and Function*, 221, 1, pp. 59–78.

Gerbella, M., Rozzi, S., Rizzolatti, G. (2017), 'The extended object-grasping network'. *Experimental Brain Research*, 235, 10, pp. 2903–2916.

Gerson, S.A., Woodward, A.L. (2014), 'Learning from their own actions: The unique effect of producing actions on infants' action understanding'. *Child Development*, 85, 1, pp. 264–277.

Gibson, W.S., Cho, S., Abulseoud, O.A., Gorny, K.R., Felmlee, J.P., Welker, K.M., Klassen, B.T., Min, H.K., Lee, K.H. (2016), 'The impact of mirth-inducing ventral striatal deep brain stimulation on functional and effective connectivity'. *Cerebral Cortex*, 27, 3, pp. 2183–2194.

Goldenberg, G. (2009), 'Apraxia and the parietal lobes'. *Neuropsychologia*, 47, 6, pp. 1449–1459.

Goldenberg, G. (2014), 'Challenging traditions in apraxia'. *Brain*, 137, 7, pp. 1858–1859.

Goldie, P. (2000), *The Emotions: A Philosophical Exploration*. Oxford University Press, Oxford.

Goldman, A.I. (2006), *Simulating Minds: The Philosophy, Psychology and Neuroscience of Mindreading*. Oxford University Press, New York.

Goldman, A.I. (2009), 'Mirroring, simulating and mindreading'. *Mind and Language*, 24, pp. 235–252.

Gothard, K.M. (2014), 'The amygdalo-motor pathways and the control of facial expressions'. *Frontiers in Neuroscience*, 19, 8, p. 43.

Gothard, K.M., Hoffman, K.L. (2010), 'Circuits of emotion in the primate brain'. In *Primate Neuroethology*, Platt, M.L., Ghazanfar, A.A. (editors). Oxford University Press, Oxford, pp. 292–315.

Grafton, S.T., Arbib, M.A., Fadiga, L., Rizzolatti, G. (1996), 'Localization of grasp representations in humans by positron emission tomography: 2. Observation compared with imagination'. *Experimental Brain Research*, 112, 1, pp. 103–111.

Gray, J.M., Young, A.W., Barker, W.A., Curtis, A., Gibson, D. (1997), 'Impaired recognition of disgust in Huntington's disease gene carriers'. *Brain*, 120, 11, pp. 2029–2038.

Graziano, M.S.A (2018), *The Space between Us. A Story of Neuroscience, Evolution, and Human Nature*. Oxford University Press, New York.

Graziano, M.S.A., Yap, G.S., Gross, C.G. (1994), 'Coding of visual space by premotor neurons'. *Science*, 266, pp. 1054–1057.

Graziano, M.S.A., Reiss, L.A.J., Gross, C.G. (1999), 'A neural representation of the location of nearby sounds'. *Nature*, 397, pp. 428–430.

Greenberg, B.D., Gabriels, L.A., Malone, D.A., Rezai, A.R., Friehs, G.M., Okun, M.S., Shapira, N.A., Foote, K.D., Cosyns, P.R., Kubu, C.S., Malloy, P.F., Salloway, S.P., Giftakis, J.E., Rise, M.T., Machado, A.G., Baker, K.B., Stypulkowski, P.H., Goodman, W.K., Rasmussen, S.A., Nuttin, B.J. (2010), 'Deep brain stimulation of the ventral internal capsule/ventral striatum for obsessive-compulsive disorder: Worldwide experience'. *Molecular Psychiatry*, 15, 1, pp. 64–79.

Greenwald, A.G. (1970), 'Sensory feedback mechanisms in performance control: With special reference to the ideo-motor mechanism'. *Psychological Review*, 77, pp. 73–99.

Grosbras, M.H., Beaton, S., Eickhoff, S.B. (2012), 'Brain regions involved in human movement perception: A quantitative voxel-based meta-analysis'. *Human Brain Mapping*, 33, 2, pp. 431–454.

Hackett, T.A. (2015), 'Anatomic organization of auditory cortex'. *Handbook of Clinical Neurology*, 129, pp. 27–53.

Hadjikhani, N., De Gelder, B. (2003), 'Seeing fearful body expressions activates the fusiform cortex and amygdala'. *Current Biology*, 13, 24, pp. 2201–2205.

Hafting, T., Fyhn, M., Molden, S., Moser, M.-B., Moser, E. (2005), 'Microstructure of a spatial map in the entorhinal cortex'. *Nature*, 436, 7052, pp. 801–806.

Hamilton, A.F.C., Wolpert, D.M., Frith, U. (2004), 'Your own action influences how you perceive another person's action'. *Current Biology*, 14, 6, pp. 493–498.

Hamilton, A.F.C., Wolpert, D.M., Frith, U., Grafton, S.T. (2006), 'Where does your own action influence your perception of another person's action in the brain?'. *NeuroImage*, 29, 2, pp. 524–535.

Hamilton, A.F.C., Brindley, R.M., Frith, U. (2007), 'Imitation and action understanding in autistic spectrum disorders: How valid is the hypothesis of a deficit in the mirror neuron system?'. *Neuropsychologia*, 45, 8, pp. 1859–1868.

Hari, R., Forss, N., Aviakainen, S., Kirverkari, S., Salenius, S., Rizzolatti, G. (1998), 'Activation of human primary motor cortex during action observation: A neuromagnetic study'. *Proceedings of National Academy of Sciences of the United States of America*, 95, pp.15061–15065.

Haslinger, B., Erhard, P., Altenmüller, E., Schroeder, U., Boecker, H., Ceballos-Baumann, A.O. (2005), 'Transmodal sensorimotor networks during action observation in professional pianists'. *Journal of Cognitive Neuroscience*, 17, 2, pp. 282–293.

Hayhoe, M., Ballard, D. (2005), 'Eye movements in natural behavior'. *Trends in Cognitive Sciences*, 9, 4, pp. 188–194

Hecht, H., Vogt, S., Prinz, W. (2001), 'Motor learning enhances perceptual judgment: A case for action-perception transfer'. *Psychological Research*, 65, 1, pp. 3–14.

Heilman, K.M., Rothi, L.J., Valenstein, E. (1982), 'Two forms of ideomotor apraxia'. *Neurology*, 32, 4, pp. 342–346.

Hennenlotter, A., Schroeder, U., Erhard, P., Castrop, F., Haslinger, B., Stoecker, D., Lange, K.W., Ceballos-Baumann, A.O. (2005), 'A common neural basis for receptive and expressive communication of pleasant facial affect'. *NeuroImage*, 26, 2, pp. 581–591.

Hickok, G. (2009), 'Eight problems for the mirror neuron theory of action understanding in monkeys and humans'. *Journal of Cognitive Neuroscience*, 21, 7, pp. 1229–1243.

Hickok, G. (2014), *The Myth of Mirror Neurons. The Real Neuroscience of Communication and Cognition.* Norton Company, New York.

Hihara, S., Taoka, M., Tanaka, M., Iriki, A. (2015), 'Visual responsiveness of neurons in the secondary somatosensory area and its surrounding parietal operculum regions in awake macaque monkeys'. *Cerebral Cortex*, 25, 11, pp. 4535–4550.

Hjortsjö, C.H. (1970), *Man's Face and Mimic Language.* Nordens Boktryekri, Malmö.

Hobson, R.P., Lee, A. (1999), 'Imitation and identification in autism'. *Journal of Child Psychology and Psychiatry and Allied Disciplines*, 40, 4, pp. 649–659.

Hobson, R.P., Hobson, J.A. (2008), 'Dissociable aspects of imitation: A study in autism'. *Journal of Experimental Child Psychology*, 101, 3, pp. 170–185.

Holstege, G.G., Mouton, L.J., Gerrits, N.M. (2004), 'Emotional motor system'. In *The Human Nervous System, Second Edition*, Paxinos, G., May, J. (editors). Elsevier Academic Press, San Diego, CA, pp. 1306–1324.

Hommel, B. (2013), 'Ideomotor action control: On the perceptual grounding of voluntary actions and agents'. In *Action Science: Foundations of an Emerging Discipline*, Prinz, W., Beisert, M., Herwig, A. (editors). MIT Press, Cambridge, MA, pp. 112–136.

Hommel, B., Müsseler, J., Aschersleben, G., Prinz, W. (2001), 'The theory of event coding (TEC): A framework for perception and action planning', *Behavioural Brain Research*, 24, 5, pp. 849–878; discussion, pp. 878–937.

Honeycutt, C.F., Kharouta, M., Perreault, E.J. (2013), 'Evidence for reticulospinal contributions to coordinated finger movements in humans'. *Journal of Neurophysiology*, 110, 7, pp. 1476–1483.

Hornung, J.P. (2003), 'The human raphe nuclei and the serotonergic system'. *Journal of Chemical Neuroanatomy*, 26, pp. 331–343.

Hutchison, W.D., Davis, K.D., Lozano, A.M., Tasker, R.R., Dostrovsky, J.O. (1999), 'Pain related neurons in the human cingulate cortex'. *Nature Neuroscience*, 2, pp. 403–405.

Hyvärinen, J. (1981), 'Regional distribution of functions in parietal association'. *Brain Research*, 206, pp. 287–303.

Iacoboni, M., Molnar-Szakacs, I., Gallese, V., Buccino, G., Mazziotta, J.C., Rizzolatti, G. (2005), 'Grasping the intentions of others with one's own mirror neuron system'. *PLoS Biology*, 3, pp. 529–535.

Iannetti, G.D., Salomons, T.V., Moayedi, M., Mouraux, A., Davis, K.D. (2013), 'Beyond metaphor: Contrasting mechanisms of social and physical pain'. *Trends in Cognitive Sciences*, 17, 8, pp. 371–378.

Ingvar, M. (1999), 'Pain and functional imaging'. *Philosophical Transactions of the Royal Society B: Biological Sciences*, 354, 1387, pp. 1347–1358.

Inman, C.S., Manns, J.R., Bijanki, K.R., Bass, D.I., Hamann, S., Drane, D.L., Fasano, R.E., Kovach, C.K., Gross, R.E., Willie, J.T. (2018), 'Direct electrical stimulation of the amygdala enhances declarative memory in humans'. *Proceedings of the National Academy of Sciences*, 115, 1, pp. 98–103.

Iriki, A., Tanaka, M., Iwamura, Y. (1996), 'Coding of modified body schema during tool use by macaque postcentral neurones'. *NeuroReport*, 7, pp. 2325–2330.

Ishai, A., Sagi, D. (1995), 'Common mechanisms of visual imagery and perception'. *Science*, 268, 5218, pp. 1772–1774.

Ishibashi, H., Hihara, S., Iriki, A. (2000), 'Acquisition and development of monkey tool-use: Behavioral and kinematic analyses'. *Canadian Journal of Physiology and Pharmacology*, 78, pp. 958–966.

Ishida, H., Nakajima, K., Inase, M., Murata, A. (2010), 'Shared mapping of own and others' bodies in visuotactile bimodal area of monkey parietal cortex'. *Journal of Cognitive Neuroscience*, 22, 1, pp. 83–96.

Isnard, J., Guénot, M., Sindou, M., Mauguière, F. (2004), 'Clinical manifestations of insular lobe seizures: A stereo-electroencephalographic study'. *Epilepsia*, 45, 9, pp. 1079–1090.

Jabbi, M., Swart, M., Keysers, C. (2007), 'Empathy for positive and negative emotions in the gustatory cortex'. *NeuroImage*, 34, 4, pp. 1744–1753.

Jackson, R.C., Warren, S., Abernethy, B. (2006), 'Anticipation skill and susceptibility to deceptive movement'. *Acta Psychologica*, 123, 3, pp. 355–371.

Jacob, P. (2009), 'The tuning-fork model of human social cognition: A critique'. *Consciousness and Cognition*, 18, 1, pp. 229–243.

Jacobs, A., Pinto, J., Shiffrar, M. (2004), 'Experience, context, and the visual perception of human movement'. *Journal of Experimental Psychology: Human Perception and Performance*, 30, 5, pp. 822–835.

Jacobs, A., Shiffrar, M. (2005), 'Walking perception by walking observers'. *Journal of Experimental Psychology: Human Perception and Performance*, 31, 1, pp. 157–169.

James, W. (1890), *The Principles of Psychology*. Henry Holt and Company, New York.

Jeannerod, M. (1994), 'The representing brain: Neural correlates of motor intention and imagery'. *Behavioral and Brain Sciences*, 17, 2, pp. 187–245.

Jeannerod, M. (2001), 'Neural simulation of action: A unifying mechanism for motor cognition'. *NeuroImage*, 14, pp. 103–109.

Jeannerod, M. (2004), 'Actions from within'. *International Journal of Sport and Exercise Psychology*, 2, pp. 376–402.

Jeannerod, M., Arbib, M.A., Rizzolatti, G., Sakata, H. (1995), 'Grasping objects: The cortical mechanisms of visuomotor transformation'. *Trends in Neuroscience*, 18, pp. 314–320.

Jeannerod, M., Decety, J. (1995), 'Mental motor imagery: A window into the representational stages of action'. *Current Opinion in Neurobiology*, 5, 6, pp. 727–732.

Jezzini, A., Caruana, F., Stoianov, I., Gallese, V., Rizzolatti, G. (2012), 'Functional organization of the insula and inner Perisylvian regions'. *Proceedings of the National Academy of Sciences*, 109, 25, pp. 10077–10082.

Jezzini, A., Rozzi, S., Borra, E., Gallese, V., Caruana, F., Gerbella, M. (2015), 'A shared neural network for emotional expression and perception: An anatomical study in the macaque monkey'. *Frontiers in Behavioral Neuroscience*, 9, p. 243.

Johansson, G. (1973), 'Visual perception of biological motion and a model for its analysis'. *Perception Psychophysics*, 14, 2, pp. 201–211.

Johansson, R.S., Westling, G., Backstrom, A., Flanagan, J.R. (2001), 'Eye-hand coordination in object manipulation'. *Journal of Neuroscience*, 21, 17, pp. 6917–6932.

Jola, C., Abedian-Amiri, A., Kuppuswamy, A., Pollick, F.E., Grosbras, M.H. (2012), 'Motor simulation without motor expertise: Enhanced corticospinal excitability in visually experienced dance spectators'. *PLoS One*, 7, 3, e33343.

Kaada, B.R., Pribram, K.H., Epstein, J. (1949), 'Respiratory and vascular responses in monkeys from temporal pole, insula, orbital surface and cingulated gyrus'. *Journal of Neurophysiology*, 12, pp. 347–356.

Kennedy, D.P., Gläscher, J., Tyszka, J.M., Adolphs, R. (2009), 'Personal space regulation by the human amygdala'. *Nature Neuroscience*, 12, 10, pp. 1226–1227.

Keysers, C., Wicker, B., Gazzola, V., Anton, J.L., Fogassi, L., Gallese, V. (2004), 'A touching sight: SII/PV activation during the observation and experience of touch'. *Neuron*, 42, 2, pp. 335–346.

Keysers, C., Gazzola, V. (2007), 'Integrating simulation and theory of mind: From self to social cognition'. *Trends in Cognitive Sciences*, 11, 5, pp. 194–196.

Khalsa, S.S., Feinstein, J.S., LI, W., Feusner, J.D., Adolphs, R., Hurlemann, R. (2016), 'Panic anxiety in humans with bilateral amygdala lesions: Pharmacological induction via cardiorespiratory interoceptive pathways'. *Journal of Neuroscience*, 36, pp. 3559–3566.

Kilner, J.M. (2011), 'More than one pathway to action understanding'. *Trends in Cognitive Sciences*, 15, 8, pp. 352–357.

Kilner, J.M., Paulignan, Y., Blakemore, S.J. (2003), 'An interference effect of observed biological movement on action'. *Current Biology*, 13, 6, pp. 522–525.

Kilner, J.M., Friston, K.J., Frith, C.D. (2007), 'Predictive coding: An account of the mirror neuron system'. *Cognitive Processing*, 8, 3, pp. 159–166.

Kilner, J.M., Frith, C.D. (2007), 'Action observation: Inferring intentions without mirror neurons'. *Current Biology*, 18, 1, R32–33.

Kilner, J.M., Kraskov, A., Lemon, R.N. (2014), 'Do monkey F5 mirror neurons show changes in firing rate during repeated observation of natural actions?'. *Journal of Neurophysiology*, 111, pp. 1214–1226.

Kipps, C.M., Duggins, A.J., McCusker, E.A., Calder, A.J. (2007), 'Disgust and happiness recognition correlate with anteroventral insula and amygdala volume respectively in preclinical Huntington's disease'. *Journal of Cognitive Neuroscience*, 19, 7, pp. 1206–1217.

Knoblich, G., Flach, R. (2001), 'Predicting the effects of actions: Interactions of perception and action'. *Psychological Science*, 12, 6, pp. 467–472.

Knoblich, G., Seigerschmidt, E., Flach, R., Prinz, W. (2002), 'Authorship effects in the prediction of handwriting strokes'. *Quarterly Journal of Experimental Psychology*, 55A, 3, pp. 1027–1046.

Kohler, E., Keysers, C., Umiltà, M.A., Fogassi, L., Gallese, V., Rizzolatti, G. (2002), 'Hearing sounds, understanding actions: Action representation in mirror neurons'. *Science*, 297, pp. 846–848.

Kosslyn, S.M. (1978), 'Measuring the visual angle of the mind's eye'. *Cognitive Psychology*, 10, 3, pp. 356–389.

Kosslyn, S.M. (1996), *Image and Brain: The Resolution of the Imagery Debate*. MIT Press, Cambridge, MA.

Kosslyn, S.M., Ball, T.M., Reiser, B.J. (1978), 'Visual images preserve metric spatial information: Evidence from studies of image scanning'. *Journal of Experimental Psychology: Human Perception and Performance*, 4, 1, pp. 47–60.

Kosslyn, S., Ganis, G., Thompson, W. (2001), 'Neural foundations of imagery'. *Nature Reviews Neuroscience*, 2, 9, pp. 635–642

Koyama, T., Kato, K., Tanaka, Y.Z., Mikami, A. (2001), 'Anterior cingulate activity during pain-avoidance and reward tasks in monkeys'. *Neuroscience Research*, 39, 4, pp. 421–430.

Koyama, T., Tanaka, Y.Z., Mikami, A. (1998), 'Nociceptive neurons in the macaque anterior cingulate activate during anticipation of pain'. *NeuroReport*, 9, 11, pp. 2663–2667

Kraskov, A., Dancause, N., Quallo, M.M., Shepherd, S., Lemon, R.N. (2009), 'Corticospinal neurons in macaque ventral premotor cortex with mirror properties: A potential mechanism for action suppression?'. *Neuron*, 64, 6, pp. 922–930.

Krolak-Salmon, P., Hénaff, M.A., Isnard, J., Tallon-Baudry, C., Guénot, M., Vighetto, A., Bertrand, O., Mauguière, F. (2003), 'An attention modulated response to disgust in human ventral anterior insula'. *Annals of Neurology*, 53, pp. 446–453.

Krolak-Salmon, P., Hénaff, M.A., Vighetto, A., Bertrand, O., Mauguière, F. (2004), 'Early amygdala reaction to fear spreading in occipital, temporal, and frontal cortex'. *Neuron*, 42, pp. 665–676.

Krolak-Salmon, P., Hénaff, M.A., Vighetto, A., Bauchet, F., Bertrand, O., Mauguière, F., Isnard, J. (2006), 'Experiencing and detecting happiness in humans: The role of the supplementary motor area'. *Annals of Neurology*, 59, 1, pp. 196–199.

Kurth, F., Zilles, K., Fox, P.T., Laird, A.R., Eickhoff, S.B. (2010), 'A link between the systems: Functional differentiation and integration within the human insula revealed by meta-analysis'. *Brain Structure Function*, 214, 5–6, pp. 519–534.

Kuypers, H. (1981), 'Anatomy of the descending pathways'. In *Handbook of Physiology*, Vol. 2., Brooks, V.B. (editor), American Physiological Society, Bethesda, pp. 597–666.

Land, M.F. (2009), 'Vision, eye movements, and natural behavior'. *Visual Neuroscience*, 26, 1, pp. 51–62.

Lanteaume, L., Khalfa, S., Régis, J., Marquis, P., Chauvel, P., Bartolomei, F. (2007), 'Emotion induction after direct intracerebral stimulations of human amygdala'. *Cerebral Cortex*, 17, 6, pp. 1307–1313.

Lanzilotto, M., Livi, A., Maranesi, M., Gerbella, M., Barz, F., Ruther, P., Fogassi, L., Rizzolatti, G., Bonini, L. (2016), 'Extending the cortical grasping network: Pre-supplementary motor neuron activity during vision and grasping of objects'. *Cerebral Cortex*, 26, 12, pp. 4435–4449.

Lanzilotto, M., Gerbella, M., Perciavalle, V., Lucchetti, C. (2017), 'Neuronal encoding of self and others' head rotation in the macaque dorsal prefrontal cortex'. *Scientific Reports*, 7, 1, p. 8571.

Lanzillotto, M., Ferroni, C.G., Livi, A., Gerbella, M., Maranesi, M., Borra, E., Passarelli, L., Gamberini, M., Fogassi, L., Bonini, L., Orban, G.A. (2019), 'Anterior intraparietal area: A hub in the observed manipulative action network'. *Cerebral Cortex*, 29, pp. 1816–1833.

Ledoux, J.E., Brown, R. (2017), 'A higher-order theory of emotional consciousness'. *Proceedings of the National Academy of Sciences*, 114, 10, E2016–E2025.

Lee, M.C., Mouraux, A., Iannetti, G.D. (2009), 'Characterizing the cortical activity through which pain emerges from nociception'. *Journal of Neuroscience*, 29, 24, pp. 7909–7916.

Lee, T.W., Josephs, O., Dolan, R.J., Critchley, H.D. (2006), 'Imitating expressions: Emotion-specific neural substrates in facial mimicry'. *Social Cognitive and Affective Neuroscience*, 1, 2, pp. 122–135.

Legrain, V., Iannetti, G.D., Plaghki, L., Mouraux, A. (2011), 'The pain matrix reloaded: A salience detection system for the body'. *Progress in Neurobiology*, 93, 1, pp. 111–124.

Leichnetz, G.R., Spencer, R.F., Hardy, S.G.P., Astruc, J. (1981), 'The pre-frontal corticotectal projection in the monkey: An anterograde and retrograde horseradish peroxidase study'. *Neuroscience*, 6, 6, pp. 1023–1041.

Lemon, R.N. (1999), 'Neural control of dexterity: What has been achieved?'. *Experimental Brain Research*, 128, pp. 6–12.

Lewis, J.W., Brefczynski, J.A., Phinney, R.E., Janik, J.J., Deyoe, E.A. (2005), 'Distinct cortical pathways for processing tool versus animal sounds'. *Journal of Neuroscience*, 25, 21, pp. 5148–5158.

Liepelt, R., Von Cramon, D.Y., Brass, M. (2008), 'How do we infer others' goals from non-stereotypic actions? The outcome of context-sensitive inferential processing in right inferior parietal and posterior temporal cortex'. *NeuroImage*, 43, 4, pp. 784–792.

Liepelt, R., Ullsperger, M., Obst, K., Spengler, S., Von Cramon, D.Y., Brass, M. (2009), 'Contextual movement constraints of others modulate motor preparation in the observer'. *Neuropsychologia*, 47, 1, pp. 268–275.

Liepmann, H. (1900), 'Das Krankheitsbild der Apraxie (Motorischen Asymbolie): auf Grund eines Falles von einseitiger Apraxie'. In *Monatsschrift für Psychiatrie und Neurologie*, 8, pp. 15–44. Translated into English as: 'The pathology of apraxia ('motor asymbolia') pursuant to a case of unilateral apraxia'. In *Neurological Classics in Modern Translation*,

Rottenberg, D.A., Hochberg, F.H. (editors), McMillan, New York, pp. 155–183.

Livi, A., Lanzilotto, M., Maranesi, M., Rizzolatti, G., Bonini, L. (2019), 'From object to action: Agent-based representations in monkey pre-supplementary motor cortex'. *Proceedings of the National Academy of Sciences*, 116, pp. 2691–2700.

Loula, F., Prasad, S., Harber, K., Shiffrar, M. (2005), 'Recognizing people from their movement'. *Journal of Experimental Psychology: Human Perception and Performance*, 31, 1, pp. 210–220.

Luppino, G., Matelli, M., Camarda, R.M., Gallese, V., Rizzolatti, G. (1991), 'Multiple representations of body movements in medial area 6 and the adjacent cingulate cortex: An intracortical microstimulation study in the macaque monkey'. *Journal of Comparative Neurology*, 311, 4, pp. 463–482.

Luppino, G., Matelli, M., Camarda, R., Rizzolatti, G. (1993), 'Corticocortical connections of area F3 (SMA-proper) and area F6 (pre-SMA) in the macaque monkey'. *Journal of Comparative Neurology*, 338, 1, pp. 1114–1140.

Luppino, G., Matelli, M., Camarda, R., Rizzolatti, G. (1994), 'Corticospinal projections from mesial frontal and cingulate areas in the monkey'. *NeuroReport*, 5, 18, pp. 2545–2548.

Luppino, G., Murata, A., Govoni, P., Matelli, M. (1999), 'Largely segregated parietofrontal connections linking rostral intraparietal cortex (areas AIP and VIP) and the ventral premotor cortex (areas F5 and F4)'. *Experimental Brain Research*, 128, pp. 181–187.

Maeda, K., Ishida, H., Nakajima, K., Inase, M., Murata, A. (2015), 'Functional properties of parietal hand manipulation-related neurons and mirror neurons responding to vision of own hand action'. *Journal of Cognitive Neuroscience*, 27, 3, pp. 560–572.

Mahon, B.Z., Caramazza, A. (2008), 'A critical look at the embodied cognition hypothesis and a new proposal for grounding conceptual content'. *Journal of Physiology Paris*, 102, 1–3, pp. 59–70.

Mahoney, M.J., Avener, M. (1977), 'Psychology of the elite athlete: An exploratory study'. *Cognitive Therapy and Research*, 1, 2, pp. 135–141.

Malloch, S., Trevarthen, C. (eds.) (2009), *Communicative Musicality. Exploring the Basis of Human Companionship*. Oxford University Press, Oxford.

Maranesi, M., Livi, A., Fogassi, L., Rizzolatti, G., Bonini, L. (2014), 'Mirror neuron activation prior to action observation in a predictable con text'. *Journal of Neuroscience*, 34, 45, pp. 14827–14832.

Maravita, A., Husain, M., Clarke, K., Driver, J. (2001), 'Reaching with a tool extends visual-tactile interactions into far space: Evidence from cross-modal extinction'. *Neuropsychologia*, 39, 6, pp. 580–585.

Mason, C.R., Gomez, J.E., Ebner, T.J. (2001), 'Hand synergies during reach-to-grasp'. *Journal of Neurophysiology*, 86, 6, pp. 2896–2910.

Matelli, M., Luppino, G., Rizzolatti, G. (1985), 'Patterns of cytochrome oxidase activity in the frontal agranular cortex of the macaque monkey'. *Behavioural Brain Research*, 18, 2, pp. 125–136.

Matelli, M., Camarda, R., Glickstein, M., Rizzolatti, G. (1986), 'Afferent and efferent projections of the inferior area 6 in the macaque monkey'. *Journal of Comparative Neurology*, 251, 3, pp. 281–298.

Matelli, M., Luppino, G., Rizzolatti, G. (1991), 'Architecture of superior and mesial area 6 and the adjacent cingulate cortex in the macaque monkey'. *Journal of Comparative Neurology*, 311, 4, pp. 445–462.

Matsunaga, M., Kawamichi, H., Koike, T., Yoshihara, K., Yoshida, Y., Takahashi, H.K., Nakagawa, E., Sadato, N. (2016), 'Structural and functional associations of the rostral anterior cingulate cortex with subjective happiness'. *NeuroImage*, 134, pp. 132–141.

Matsuzaka, Y., Aizawa, H., Tanji, J. (1992), 'A motor area rostral to the supplementary motor area (presupplementary motor area) in the monkey: Neuronal activity during a learned motor task'. *Journal of Neurophysiology*, 68, 3, pp. 653–662.

May, P.J. (2006), 'The mammalian superior colliculus: Laminar structure and connections'. *Progress in Brain Research*, 1, 51, pp. 321–378.

Mayer, J.S., Bittner, R.A., Nikolić, D., Bledowski, C., Goebel, R., Linden, D.E.J. (2007), 'Common neural substrates for visual working memory and attention'. *NeuroImage*, 36, 2, pp. 441–453.

Meletti, S., Tassi, L., Mai, R., Fini, N., Tassinari, C.A., Russo, G.L. (2006), 'Emotions induced by intracerebral electrical stimulation of the temporal lobe'. *Epilepsia*, 5, pp. 47–51.

Melzack, R. (2001), 'Pain and the neuromatrix in the brain'. *Journal of Dental Education*, 65, 12, pp. 1378–1382.

Melzack, R. (2005), 'Evolution of the neuromatrix theory of pain'. *Pain Practice: The Official Journal of World Institute of Pain*, 5, 2, pp. 85–94.

Méndez-Bértolo, C., Moratti, S., Toledano, R., Lopez-Sosa, F., Martínez-Alvarez, R., Mah, Y.H., Vuilleumier, P., Gil-Nagel, A., Strange, B.A. (2016), 'A fast pathway for fear in human amygdala'. *Nature Neuroscience*, 19, 8, pp. 1041–1049.

Mercier, C., Reilly, K., Vargas, C.D., Aballea, A., Sirigu, A. (2006), 'Mapping phantom movement representations in the motor cortex of amputees'. *Brain*, 129, 8, pp. 2202–2210.

Mesulam, M.M., Mufson, E.J. (1982a), 'Insula of the old-world monkey: I. Architectonics in the insulo-orbito-temporal component of the paralimbic brain'. *Journal of Comparative Neurology*, 212, pp. 1–22.

Mesulam, M.M., Mufson, E.J. (1982b), 'Insula of the old world monkey: III. Efferent cortical output and comments on function'. *Journal of Comparative Neurology*, 212, pp. 38–52.

Miall, R.C., Stanley, J., Todhunter, S., Levick, C., Lindo, S., Miall, J.D. (2006), 'Performing hand actions assists the visual discrimination of similar hand postures'. *Neuropsychologia*, 44, 6, pp. 966–976.

Michael, J., Sandberg, K., Skewes, J., Wolf, T., Blicher, J., Overgaard, M., Frith, C.D. (2014), 'Continuous theta-burst stimulation demonstrates a causal role of premotor homunculus in action understanding'. *Psychological Science*, 25, 4, pp. 963–972.

Miyashita, Y. (1988), 'Neuronal correlate of visual associative long-term memory in the primate temporal cortex'. *Nature*, 335, pp. 817–820.

Moga, M.M., Gray, T.S. (1985), 'Evidence for corticotropin-releasing factor, neurotensin, and somatostatin in the neural pathway from the central nucleus of the amygdala to the parabrachial nucleus'. *Journal of Comparative Neurology*, 241, 3, pp. 275–284.

Molenberghs, P., Cunnington, R., Mattingley, J.B. (2012), 'Brain regions with mirror properties: A meta-analysis of 125 human fMRI studies'. *Neuroscience and Biobehavioral Reviews*, 36, 1, pp. 341–349.

Mooney, R. (2014), 'Auditory-vocal mirroring in songbirds'. *Philosophical Transactions of the Royal Society B: Biological Sciences*, 369, 1644, 20130179.

Morecraft, R.J., Louie, J.L., Herrick, J.L., Stilwell-Morecraft, K.S. (2001), 'Cortical innervation of the facial nucleus in the non-human primate: A new interpretation of the effects of stroke and related subtotal brain trauma on the muscles of facial expression'. *Brain*, 124, 1, pp. 176–208.

Morecraft, R.J., Stilwell-Morecraft, K.S., Cipolloni, P.B., GE, J., Mcneal, D.W., Pandya, D.N. (2012), 'Cytoarchitecture and cortical connections of the anterior cingulate and adjacent somatomotor fields in the rhesus monkey'. *Brain Research Bulletin*, 87, 4–5, pp. 457–497.

Moro, V., Urgesi, C., Pernigo, S., Lanteri, P., Pazzaglia, M., Aglioti, S.M. (2008), 'The neural basis of body form and body action agnosia'. *Neuron*, 60, 2, pp. 235–246.

Morris, J.S., Frith, C.D., Perrett, D.I., Rowland, D., Young, A.W., Calder, A.J., Dolan, R.J. (1996), 'A differential neural response in the human amygdala to fearful and happy facial expressions'. *Nature*, 383, 6603, pp. 812–815.

Morris, J.S., Ohman, A. (1999), 'A subcortical pathway to the right amygdala mediating 'unseen' fear'. *Neurobiology*, 96, pp. 1680–1685.

Moser, E.I., Kropf, E., Moser, M.B. (2008), 'Place cells, grid cells, and the brain's spatial representation system'. *Annual Review of Neuroscience*, 31, pp. 69–89.

Moser, E.I., Moser, M.-B., McNaughton, B.L. (2017), 'Spatial representation in the hippocampal formation: A history'. *Nature Neuroscience*, 20, pp. 1448–1464.

Motta, S.C., Goto, M., Gouveia, F.V., Baldo, M.V.C., Canteras, N.S., Swanson, L.W. (2009), 'Dissecting the brain's fear system reveals the hypothalamus is critical for responding in subordinate conspecific intruders'. *Proceedings of the National Academy of Sciences*, 106, 12, pp. 4870–4875.

Mountcastle, V.B. (1995), 'The parietal system and some higher brain functions'. *Cerebral Cortex*, 5, 5, pp. 377–390.

Mouraux, A., Diukova, A., Lee, M.C., Wise, R.G., Iannetti, G.D. (2011), 'A multisensory investigation of the functional significance of the "pain matrix"'. *NeuroImage*, 54, 3, pp. 2237–2249.

Mufson, E.J., Mesulam, M.M. (1982), 'Insula of the old-world monkey. II: Afferent cortical output and comments on the claustrum'. *Journal of Comparative Neurology*, 212, pp. 23–37.

Mukamel, R., Ekstrom, A.D., Kaplan, J., Iacoboni, M., Fried, I. (2010), 'Single-neuron responses in humans during execution and observation of actions'. *Current Biology*, 20, 8, pp. 750–756.

Müller-Preuss, P., Jürgens, U. (1976), 'Projections from the 'cingular' vocalization area in the squirrel monkey'. *Brain Research*, 103, 1, pp. 29–43.

Murata, A., Fadiga, L., Fogassi, L., Gallese, V., Raos, V., Rizzolatti, G. (1997), 'Object representation in the ventral premotor cortex (Area F5) of the monkey'. *Journal of Neurophysiology*, 78, 4, pp. 2226–2230.

Murata, A., Gallese, V., Luppino, G., Kaseda, M., Sakata, H. (2000), 'Selectivity for the shape, size, and orientation of objects for grasping in neurons of monkey parietal area AIP'. *Journal of Neurophysiology*, 83, 5, pp. 2580–2601.

Murray, R.J., Brosch, T., Sander, D. (2014), 'The functional profile of the human amygdala in affective processing: Insights from intracranial recordings'. *Cortex*, 60, pp. 10–33.

Müsseler, J., Hommel, B. (1997), 'Blindness to response-compatible stimuli'. *Journal of Experimental Psychology: Human Perception and Performance*, 23, 3, pp. 861–872.

Müsseler, J., Steininger, S., Wühr, P. (2001), 'Can actions affect perceptual processing?'. *Quarterly Journal of Experimental Psychology Section A: Human Experimental Psychology*, 54, 1, pp. 137–154.

Naor, N., Shamay-Tsoory, S.G., Sheppes, G., Okon-Singer, H. (2018), 'The impact of empathy and reappraisal on emotional intensity recognition'. *Cognition and Emotion*, 32, 5, pp. 972–987.

Nee, D.E., Wager, T.D., Jonides, J. (2007), 'Interference resolution: Insights from a meta–analysis of neuroimaging tasks'. *Cognitive, Affective and Behavioral Neuroscience*, 7, 1, pp. 1–17.

Nelissen, K., Luppino, G., Vanduffel, W., Rizzolatti, G., Orban, G.A. (2005), 'Neuroscience: Observing others: Multiple action representation in the frontal lobe'. *Science*, 310, 5746, pp. 332–336.

Neppi-Mòdona, M., Rabuffetti, M., Folegatti, A., Ricci, R., Spinazzola, L., Schiavone, F., Ferrarin, M., Berti, A. (2007), 'Bisecting lines with different tools in right brain damaged patients: The role of action programming and sensory feedback in modulating spatial remapping'. *Cortex*, 43, 3, pp. 397–410.

Niedenthal, P.M., Mermillod, M., Maringer, M., Hess, U. (2010), 'The simulation of smiles (SIMS) model: Embodied simulation and the meaning of facial expression'. *Behavioral and Brain Sciences*, 33, pp. 417–480.

Nikolajsen, L., Jensen, T.S. (2006), 'Phantom limb'. In *Textbook of Pain*, 5th edition, McMahon, S.B., Koltzenburg, M. (editors), Churchill Livingstone, Edinburgh, pp. 961–971.

Nishimura, A., Yokosawa, K. (2010), 'Response-specifying cue for action interferes with perception of feature-sharing stimuli'. *Quarterly Journal of Experimental Psychology*, 63, 6, pp. 1150–1167.

Nishitani, N., Hari, R. (2000), 'Temporal dynamics of cortical representation for action'. *Proceedings of National Academy of Sciences*, 97, pp. 913–918.

O'Keefe, J., Nadel, L. (1978), *The Hippocampus as a Cognitive Map*. Oxford University Press, Oxford.

Olson, I.R., Plotzker, A., Ezzyat, Y. (2007), 'The enigmatic temporal pole: A review of findings on social and emotional processing'. *Brain*, 7, pp. 1718–1731.

Omer, D.B., Maimon, S.R., Las, L., Ulanovsky, N. (2018), 'Social place-cells in the bat hippocampus'. *Science*, 359, 6372, pp. 218–224.

Öngür, D., An, X., Price, J.L. (1998), 'Prefrontal cortical projections to the hypothalamus in macaque monkeys'. *Journal of Comparative Neurology*, 401, 4, pp. 480–505.

Ortigue, S., Sinigaglia, C., Rizzolatti, G., Grafton, S.T. (2010), 'Understanding actions of others: The electrodynamics of the left and right hemispheres. A high-density EEG neuroimaging study'. *PLoS One*, 5, 8, e12160.

Page, J.W., Duhamel, P., Crognale, M.A. (2011), 'ERP evidence of visualization at early stages of visual processing'. *Brain and Cognition*, 75, 2, pp. 141–146.

Palomero-Gallagher, N., Eickhoff, S.B., Hoffstaedter, F., Schleicher, A., Mohlberg, H., Vogt, B.A., Amunts, K., Zilles, K. (2015), 'Functional organization of human subgenual cortical areas: Relationship between architectonical segregation and connectional heterogeneity'. *NeuroImage*, 115, pp. 177–190.

Palomero-Gallagher, N., Mohlberg, H., Zilles, K., Vogt, B.A. (2008), 'Cytology and receptor architecture of human anterior cingulate cortex'. *Journal of Comparative Neurology*, 508, 6, pp. 906–926.

Palomero-Gallagher, N., Vogt, B.A., Schleicher, A., Mayberg, H.S., Zilles, K. (2009), 'Receptor architecture of human cingulate cortex: Evaluation of the four-region neurobiological model'. *Human Brain Mapping*, 30, 8, pp. 2336–2355.

Panasiti, M.S., Pavone, E.F., Aglioti, S.M. (2016), 'Electrocortical signatures of detecting errors in the actions of others: An EEG study in pianists, non-pianist musicians and musically naïve people'. *Neuroscience*, 318, pp. 104–113.

Pandya, D.N., Van Hoesen, G.W., Mesulam, M.M. (1981), 'Efferent connections of the cingulate gyrus in the rhesus monkey'. *Experimental Brain Research*, 42, 3–4, pp. 319–330.

Pani, P., Theys, T., Romero, M.C., Janssen, P. (2014), 'Grasping execution and grasping observation activity of single neurons in the macaque anterior intraparietal area'. *Journal of Cognitive Neuroscience*, 26, 10, pp. 2342–2355.

Panksepp, J. (1998), *Affective Neuroscience: The Foundations of Human and Animal Emotions*. Oxford University Press, Oxford.

Panksepp, J., Biven, L. (2012), *The Archaeology of Mind: Neuroevolutionary Origins of Human Emotion*. W.W. Norton and Co., New York.

Papadourakis, V., Raos, V. (2018), 'Neurons in the macaque dorsal premotor cortex respond to execution and observation of actions'. *Cerebral Cortex*, 29, 10, pp. 4017–4461.

Papagno, C., Pisoni, A., Mattavelli, G., Casarotti, A., Comi, A., Fumagalli, F., Vernice, M., Fava, E., Riva, M., Bello, L. (2016), 'Specific disgust processing in the left insula: New evidence from direct electrical stimulation'. *Neuropsychologia*, 84, pp. 29–35.

Parsons, L.M. (1994), 'Temporal and kinematic properties of motor behavior reflected in mentally simulated action'. *Journal of Experimental Psychology: Human Perception and Performance*, 20, 4, pp. 709–730.

Pazzaglia, M., Pizzamiglio, L., Pes, E., Aglioti, S.M. (2008), 'The sound of actions in apraxia'. *Current Biology*, 18, 22, pp. 1766–1772.

Pazzaglia, M., Smania, N., Corato, E., Aglioti, S.M., Psicologia, D., Sapienza, L., Lucia, F.S. (2008), 'Neural underpinnings of gesture discrimination in patients with limb apraxia'. *Journal of Neuroscience*, 28, 12, pp. 3030–3041.

Pearson, J., Clifford, C.W.G., Tong, F. (2008), 'The functional impact of mental imagery on conscious perception'. *Current Biology*, 18, 13, pp. 982–986.

Peelen, M.V., Wiggett, A.J., Downing, P.E. (2006), 'Patterns of fMRI activity dissociate overlapping functional brain areas that respond to biological motion'. *Neuron*, 49, 6, pp. 815–822.

Peeters, R., Simone, L., Nelissen, K., Fabbri-Destro, M., Vanduffel, W., Rizzolatti, G., Orban, G.A. (2009), 'The representation of tool use in humans and monkeys: Common and uniquely human features'. *Journal of Neuroscience*, 29, 37, pp. 11523–11539.

Pegna, A.J., Petit, L., Caldara-Schnetzer, A.S., Khateb, A., Annoni, J.M., Sztajzel, R., Landis, T. (2001), 'So near yet so far: Neglect in far or near space depends on tool use'. *Annals of Neurology*, 50, 6, pp. 820–822.

Penfield, W., Faulk, M.E. (1955), 'The insula: Further observations on its function'. *Brain*, 78, pp. 445–470.

Pernet, C.R., McAleer, P., Latinus, M., Gorgolewski, K.J., Charest, I., Bestelmeyer, P.E.G., Watson, R.H., Fleming, D., Crabbe, F., Valdes-Sosa, M., Belin, P. (2015), The human voice areas: Spatial organization and inter-individual variability in temporal and extra-temporal cortices. *NeuroImage*, 119, pp. 164–174.

Perrett, D.I., Smith, P.A.J., Potter, D.D., Mistlin, A.J., Head, A.S., Milner, A.D., Jeeves, M.A. (1985), 'Visual cells in the temporal cortex sensitive to face view and gaze direction'. *Proceedings of the Royal Society of London B: Biological Sciences*, 223, 1232, pp. 293–317.

Perrett, D.I., Harries, M.H, Bevan, R., Thomas, S., Benson, P.J., Mistlin, A.J., Chitty, A.J., Hietanen, J.K., Ortega, J.E. (1989), 'Frameworks of analysis for the neural representation of animate objects and actions'. *Journal of Experimental Biology*, 146, pp. 87–113.

Perrett, D.I., Mistlin, A.J., Harries, M.H., Chitty, A.J (1990), 'Understanding the visual appearance and consequence of hand actions'. In *Vision and Action: The Control of Grasping*, Goodale, M.A. (editor), Ablex, Norwood, pp. 163–180.

Petrides, M. (2007), 'The orbitofrontal cortex: novelty, deviation from expectation, and memory'. *Proceedings of National Academy of Sciences*, 1121, pp. 33–53

Peyron, R., Laurent, B., García-Larrea, L. (2000), 'Functional imaging of brain responses to pain. A review and meta-analysis'. *Neurophysiologie Clinique*, 30, 5, pp. 263–288.

Phillips, M.L., Young, A.W., Senior, C., Brammer, M., Andrew, C., Calder, A.J., Bullmore, E.T., Perrett, D.I., Rowland, D., William, S.C., Gray, J.A., David, A.S. (1997), 'A specific neural substrate for perceiving facial expressions of disgust'. *Nature*, 389, pp. 495–498.

Phillips, M.L., Young, A.W., Scott, S.K., Calder, A.J., Andrew, C., Giampietro, V., William, S.C., Bullmore, E.T., Brammer, M., Gray, J.A. (1998), 'Neural responses to facial and vocal expressions of fear and disgust'. *Proceedings of the Royal Society of London B: Biological Sciences*, 265, pp. 1089–1817.

Picard, N., Strick, P.L. (1996), 'Motor areas of the medial wall: a review of their location and functional activation'. *Cerebral Cortex*, 6, pp. 342–353.

Pobric, G., Hamilton, A.F.C. (2006), 'Action understanding requires the left inferior frontal cortex'. *Current Biology*, 16, 5, pp. 524–529.

Porrino, L.J., Goldman-Rakic, P.S. (1982), 'Brainstem innervation of prefrontal and anterior cingulate cortex in the rhesus monkey revealed by retrograde transport of HRP'. *Journal of Comparative Neurology*, 205, 1, pp. 63–76.

Porro, C.A. (2003), 'Functional imaging and pain: Behavior, perception, and modulation'. *Neuroscientist*, 9, 5, pp. 354–369.

Prasad, S., Shiffrar, M. (2009), 'Viewpoint and the recognition of people from their movements'. *Journal of Experimental Psychology: Human Perception and Performance*, 35, 1, pp. 39–49.

Prather, J.F., Peters, S., Nowicki, S., Mooney, R. (2008), 'Precise auditory-vocal mirroring in neurons for learned vocal communication'. *Nature*, 451, 7176, pp. 305–310.

Price, J.L., Russchen, F.T., Amaral, D.G. (1987), 'The limbic region. II: The amygdaloid complex'. In *Handbook of Chemical Neuroanatomy*, Bjorkland, A., Hokfelt, T., Swanson, L. (editors), Elsevier, Amsterdam, pp. 279–381.

Prinz, W. (1987), 'Ideo-motor action'. In *Perspectives on Perception and Action*, Heuer, H., Sanders, A.F. (editors), Lawrence Erlbaum, Hillsdale, pp. 47–76.

Prinz, W. (1990), 'A common coding approach to perception and action'. In *Relationships between Perception and Action*, Neumann, O., Prinz, W. (editors), Springer, Berlin-Heidelberg-New York, pp. 167–201.

Rainville, P. (2002), 'Brain mechanisms of pain affect and pain modulation'. *Current Opinion in Neurobiology*, 12, pp. 195–204.

Rainville, P., Duncan, G.H., Price, D.D., Carrier, B., Bushnell, M.C. (1997), 'Pain affect encoded in human anterior cingulate but not somatosensory cortex'. *Science*, 277, 5328, pp. 968–971.

Ramsey, R., Cumming, J., Eastough, D., Edwards, M.G. (2010), 'Incongruent imagery interferes with action initiation'. *Brain and Cognition*, 74, 3, pp. 249–254.

Repp, B.H., Knoblich, G. (2007), 'Action can affect auditory perception: Short report'. *Psychological Science*, 18, 1, pp. 6–7.

Repp, B.H., Knoblich, G. (2009), 'Performed or observed keyboard actions affect pianists' judgements of relative pitch'. *Quarterly Journal of Experimental Psychology*, 62, 11, pp. 2156–2170.

Ricciardi, E., Bonino, D., Sani, L., Vecchi, T., Guazzelli, M., Haxby, J.V., Fadiga, L., Pietrini, P. (2009), 'Do we really need vision? How blind people 'see' the actions of others'. *Journal of Neuroscience*, 29, 31, pp. 9719–9724.

Ricciardi, E., Menicagli, D., Leo, A., Costantini, M., Pietrini, P., Sinigaglia, C. (2017), 'Peripersonal space representation develops independently from visual experience'. *Scientific Reports*, 7, 1, 17673.

Rizzolatti, G., Camarda, R., Fogassi, L., Gentilucci, M., Luppino, G., Matelli, M. (1988), 'Functional organization of inferior area 6 in the macaque monkey. II: Area F5 and the control of distal movements'. *Experimental Brain Research*, 71, pp. 491–507.

Rizzolatti, G., Fadiga, L., Gallese, V., Fogassi, L. (1996), 'Premotor cortex and the recognition of motor actions'. *Cognitive Brain Research*, 3, p. 131–141.

Rizzolatti, G., Fadiga, L., Matelli, M., Bettinardi, V., Paulesu, E., Perani, D., Fazio, F. (1996), 'Localization of grasp representations in humans by PET. 1: Observation versus execution'. *Experimental Brain Research*, 111, 2, pp. 246–252.

Rizzolatti, G., Fadiga, L., Fogassi, L., Gallese, V. (1997), 'The space around us'. *Science*, 277, pp. 190–191.

Rizzolatti, G., Fogassi, L., Gallese, V. (2001), 'Neurophysiological mechanisms underlying the understanding and imitation of action'. *Nature Reviews Neuroscience*, 2, pp. 661–670.

Rizzolatti, G., Sinigaglia, C. (2008), *Mirrors in the Brain: How Our Minds Share Actions, Emotions.* Oxford University Press, Oxford.

Rizzolatti, G., Sinigaglia, C. (2010), 'The functional role of the parieto-frontal mirror circuit: Interpretations and misinterpretations'. *Nature Reviews Neuroscience*, 11, 4, pp. 264–274.

Rizzolatti, G., Sinigaglia, C. (2013), 'Understanding action from the inside'. In *Action Science. Foundations of an Emerging Discipline*, Prinz, W., Beisert, M., Herwig, A. (editors), MIT Press, Cambridge, MA, pp. 200–227.

Rizzolatti, G., Cattaneo, L., Fabbri-Destro, M., Rozzi, S. (2014), 'Cortical mechanisms underlying the organization of goal-directed actions and mirror neuron-based action understanding'. *Physiological Reviews*, 94, 2, pp. 655–706.

Rizzolatti, G., Sinigaglia, C. (2016), 'The mirror mechanism: A basic principle of brain function'. *Nature Reviews Neuroscience*, 17, 12, pp. 757–765.

Rochat, P. (1999) (editor), *Early Social Cognition*. Erlbaum, Mahwah, NJ.

Rochat, P. (2009), *Others in Mind: Social Origins of Self-Consciousness.* Cambridge University Press, Cambridge.

Rochat, M.J., Caruana, F., Jezzini, A., Escola, L., Intskirveli, I., Grammont, F., Gallese, V., Rizzolatti, G., Umiltà, M.A. (2010), 'Responses of mirror neurons in area F5 to hand and tool grasping observation'. *Experimental Brain Research*, 204, 4, pp. 605–616.

Rochat, M.J., Veroni, V., Bruschweiler-Stern, N., Pieraccini, C., Bonnet-Brilhault, F., Barthélémy, C., Malvy, J., Sinigaglia, C., Stern, D.N., Rizzolatti, G. (2013), 'Impaired vitality form recognition in autism'. *Neuropsychologia*, 51, 10, pp. 1918–1924.

Ross, E.D. (1996), 'Hemispheric specialization for emotions, affective aspects of language and communication and the cognitive control of display behaviors in humans'. In *The Emotional Motor System*, Holstege, G., Bandler, R., Saper, C.B. (editors), *Progress in Brain Research*, Vol. 107. Elsevier Science, pp. 581–594.

Rothi, L.J.G., Heilman, K.M., Watson, R.T. (1985), 'Pantomime comprehension and ideomotor apraxia'. *Journal of Neurology Neurosurgery and Psychiatry*, 48, 3, pp. 207–210.

Rotman, G., Troje, N.F., Johansson, R.S., Flanagan, J.R. (2006), 'Eye movements when observing predictable and unpredictable actions'. *Journal of Neurophysiology*, 96, 3, pp. 1358–1369.

Rozin, R., Haidt, J., McCauley, C.R. (2000), 'Disgust'. In *Handbook of Emotions*, 2nd edition, Lewis, M., Haviland-Jones, J.M. (editors), Guilford Press, New York, pp. 637–653.

Rozzi, S., Calzavara, R., Belmalih, A., Borra, E., Gregoriou, G.G., Matelli, M., Luppino, G. (2006), 'Cortical connections of the inferior parietal cortical convexity of the macaque monkey'. *Cerebral Cortex*, 16, 10, pp. 1389–1417.

Rozzi, S., Ferrari, P.F., Bonini, L., Rizzolatti, G., Fogassi, L. (2008), 'Functional organization of inferior parietal lobule convexity in the macaque monkey: Electrophysiological characterization of motor, sensory and mirror responses and their correlation with cytoarchitectonic areas'. *European Journal of Neuroscience*, 28, 8, pp. 1569–1588.

Sakata, H., Taira, M., Murata, A., Mine, S. (1995), 'Neural mechanisms of visual guidance of hand action in the parietal cortex of the monkey'. *Cerebral Cortex*, 5, 5, pp. 429–438.

Sakay, K., Miyashita, Y. (1991), 'Neural organization for long-term memory of paired associates'. *Nature*, 354, pp. 152–155.

Santello, M., Flanders, M., Soechting, J.F. (2002), 'Patterns of hand motion during grasping and the influence of sensory guidance'. *Journal of Neuroscience*, 22, 4, pp. 1426–1435.

Sato, W., Yoshikawa, S., Kochiyama, T., Matsumura, M. (2004), 'The amygdala processes the emotional significance of facial expressions: An fMRI investigation using the interaction between expression and face direction'. *NeuroImage*, 22, pp. 1006–1013.

Sato, W., Kochiyama, T., Uono, S., Matsuda, K., Usui, K., Inoue, Y., Toichi, M. (2011), 'Rapid amygdala gamma oscillations in response to fearful facial expressions'. *Neuropsychologia*, 49, 4, pp. 612–617.

Satow, T., Usui, K., Matsuhashi, M., Yamamoto, J., Begum, T., Shibasaki, H., Ikeda, A., Mikuni, N., Miyamoto, S., Hashimoto, N. (2003), 'Mirth and laughter arising from human temporal cortex'. *Journal of Neurology, Neurosurgery, and Psychiatry*, 74, 7, pp. 1004–1005.

Saxe, R., Kanwisher, N. (2003), 'People thinking about thinking people: The role of the temporo-parietal junction in "theory of mind"'. *Social Neuroscience: Key Readings*, 19, pp. 171–182.

Saxe, R., Xiao, D.K., Kovacs, G., Perrett, D.I., Kanwisher, N. (2004), 'A region of right posterior superior temporal sulcus responds to observed intentional actions'. *Neuropsychologia*, 42, 11, pp. 1435–1446.

Scarantino, A. (2016), 'The philosophy of emotions and its impact on affective science'. In *Handbook of Emotions*, 4th edition, Lewis, M., Haviland-Jones, J., Barrett, L.F. (editors), Guilford University Press, New York, pp. 3–48.

Schmitt, J.J., Janszky, J., Woermann, F., Tuxhorn, I., Ebner, A. (2006), 'Laughter and the mesial and lateral premotor cortex'. *Epilepsy and Behavior*, 8, 4, pp. 773–775.

Schwartz, G.E., Ahern, G.L., Brown, S.-L. (1979), 'Lateralized facial muscle response to positive and negative emotional stimuli'. *Psycho-physiology*, 16, 6, pp. 561–571.

Seltzer, B., Pandya, D.N. (1991), Post-rolandic cortical projections of the superior temporal sulcus in the rhesus monkey. *Journal of Comparative Neurology*, 312, 4, pp. 625–640.

Serino, A., De Filippo, L., Casavecchia, C., Coccia, M., Shiffrar, M., Làdavas, E. (2009), 'Lesions to the motor system affect action perception'. *Journal of Cognitive Neuroscience*, 22, 3, pp. 413–426.

Shackman, A.J., Salomons, T.V., Slagter, H.A., Fox, A.S., Winter, J.J., Davidson, R.J. (2011), 'The integration of negative affect, pain and cognitive control in the cingulate cortex'. *Nature Reviews Neuroscience*, 12, pp. 154–167.

Shamay-Tsoory, S.G. (2011), 'The neural bases for empathy'. *Neuroscientist*, 17, 1, pp. 18–24.

Shepherd, S.V., Klein, J.T., Deaner, R.O., Platt, M.L. (2009), 'Mirroring of attention by neurons in macaque parietal cortex'. *Proceedings of the National Academy of Sciences*, 106, 23, pp. 9489–9494.

Shiffrar, M. (2011), 'People watching: Visual, motor, and social processes in the perception of human movement'. *Wiley Interdisciplinary Reviews: Cognitive Science*, 2, 1, pp. 68–78.

Shiffrar, M., Freyd, J.J. (1990), 'Apparent motion of the human body'. *Psychological Science*, 1, 4, pp. 257–264.

Shiffrar, M., Heinen, T. (2011), 'Athletic ability changes action perception: Embodiment in the visual perception of human movement'. *Zeitschrift für Sportpsychologie (German Journal of Sport Psychology)*, 17, 4, pp. 1–13.

Showers, M.J.C., Lauer, E.W. (1961), 'Somatovisceral motor patterns in the insula'. *Journal of Comparative Neurology*, 117, pp. 107–115.

Simone, L., Rozzi, S., Bimbi, M., Fogassi, L. (2015), 'Movement-related activity during goal-directed hand actions in the monkey ventrolateral pre-frontal cortex'. *European Journal of Neuroscience*, 42, pp. 2882–2894.

Simone, L., Bimbi, M., Rodà, F., Fogassi, L., Rozzi, S. (2017), 'Action observation activates neurons of the monkey ventrolateral prefrontal cortex'. *Scientific Reports*, 7, 44378.

Singer, T., Seymur, B., O'Doherty, J., Kaube, H., Dolan, R.J., Frith, C.D. (2004), 'Empathy for pain involves the affective but not the sensory components of pain'. *Science*, 303, pp. 1157–1162.

Sinigaglia, C., Rizzolatti, G. (2011), 'Through the looking glass: Self and others'. *Consciousness and Cognition*, 20, 1, pp. 64–74.

Sinigaglia, C., Butterfill, S.A. (2015a), 'Motor representation in goal ascription'. In *Conceptual and Interactive Embodiment. Foundations of Embodied*

Cognition, vol. II, Fischer, M.H., Coello, Y. (editors), Routledge, Oxford, pp. 149–164.

Sinigaglia, C., Butterfill, S.A. (2015b), 'On a puzzle about relations between thought, experience and the motoric'. *Synthese*, 192, 6, pp. 1923–1936.

Sinigaglia, C., Rizzolatti, G. (2015), 'The space of mirrors'. In Ferrari, P.F., Rizzolatti, G. (editors), *New Frontiers in Mirror Neurons Research*. Oxford University Press, New York, pp. 331–347.

Sinigaglia, C., Butterfill, S. (2020), 'Motor representation and action experience in joint action'. In *Minimal Cooperation and Shared Agency*, Fiebich, A. (editor), pp. 181–194, Springer, Cham, Switzerland.

Solstad, T., Boccara, C.N., Kropff, E., Moser, M.B., Moser, E.I. (2008), 'Representation of geometric borders in the entorhinal cortex'. *Science*, 322, 5909, pp. 1865–1868.

Sommerville, J.A., Woodward, A.L., Needham, A. (2005), 'Action experience alters 3-month-old infants' perception of others' actions'. *Cognition*, 96, 1, B1–11.

Sörös, P., Marmurek, J., Tam, F., Baker, N., Staines, W.R., Graham, S.J. (2007), 'Functional MRI of working memory and selective attention in vibrotactile frequency discrimination'. *BMC Neuroscience*, 8, p. 48.

Sowden, S., Catmur, C. (2015), 'The role of the right temporoparietal junction in the control of imitation'. *Cerebral Cortex*, 25, 4, pp. 1107–1113.

Sperli, F., Spinelli, L., Pollo, C., Seeck, M. (2006), 'Contralateral smile and laughter, but no mirth, induced by electrical stimulation of the cingulate cortex'. *Epilepsia*, 47, 2, pp. 440–443.

Sprengelmeyer, R., Young, A.W., Calder, A.J., Karnat, A., Lange, H., Hömberg, V., Perrett, D.I., Rowland, D. (1996), 'Loss of disgust: Perception of faces and emotions in Huntington's disease'. *Brain*, 119, 5, pp. 1647–1665.

Sprengelmeyer, R., Rausch, M., Eysel, U.T., Przuntek, H. (1998), 'Neural structures associated with recognition of facial expressions of basic emotions'. *Proceedings of the Royal Society B: Biological Sciences*, 265, 1409, pp. 1927–1931.

Sprengelmeyer, R., Young, A.W., Schroeder, U., Grossenbacher, P.G., Federlein, J., Büttner, T., Przuntek, H. (1999), 'Knowing no fear'. *Proceedings of the Royal Society B: Biological Sciences*, 266, 1437, pp. 2451–2456.

Stefanacci, L., Amaral, D.G. (2000), 'Topographic organization of cortical inputs to the lateral nucleus of the macaque monkey amygdala: A retrograde tracing study'. *Journal of Comparative Neurology*, 421, 1, pp. 52–79.

Stern, D. (1985), *The Interpersonal World of the Infant*. Basic Books, New York.

Stern, D. (2004), *The Present Moment in Psychotherapy and Everyday Life*. W.W. Norton & Co. New York.

Stern, D. (2010), *Forms of Vitality: Exploring Dynamic Experience in Psychology, the Arts, Psychotherapy, and Development*. Oxford University Press, New York.

Stevens, J.A., Fonlupt, P., Shiffrar, M., Decety, J. (2000), 'New aspects of motion perception: Selective neural encoding of apparent human movements'. *NeuroReport*, 11, 1, pp. 109–115.

Stock, A., Stock, C. (2004), 'A short history of ideo-motor action'. *Psychological Research*, 68, 2–3, pp. 176–188.

Strafella, A.P., Paus, T. (2000), 'Modulation of cortical excitability during action observation: A transcranial magnetic stimulation study'. *NeuroReport*, 11, pp. 2289–2292.

Suzuki, W., Banno, T., Miyakawa, N., Abe, H., Goda, N., Ichinohe, N. (2015), 'Mirror neurons in a new world monkey, common marmoset'. *Frontiers in Neuroscience*, 9, p. 459.

Suzuki, W., Tani, T., Banno, T., Miyakawa, N., Abe, H., Ichinohe, N. (2015), 'Functional columns in superior temporal sulcus areas of the common marmoset'. *NeuroReport*, 26, 18, pp. 1133–1139.

Szameitat, D.P., Kreifelts, B., Alter, K., Szameitat, A.J., Sterr, A., Grodd, W., Wildgruber, D. (2010), 'It is not always tickling: Distinct cerebral responses during perception of different laughter types'. *NeuroImage*, 53, 4, pp. 1264–1271.

Taira, M., Mine, S., Georgopulos, A.P., Murata, A., Sakata, H. (1990), 'Parietal cortex neurons of the monkey related to the visual guidance of hand movement'. *Experimental Brain Research*, 83, pp. 29–36.

Talairach, J., Bancaud, J., Geier, S., Bordas-Ferrer, M., Bonis, A., Szikla, G., Rusu, M. (1973), 'The cingulate gyrus and human behaviour'. *Electroencephalography and Clinical Neurophysiology*, 34, 1, pp. 45–52.

Tessari, A., Canessa, N., Ukmar, M., Rumiati, R.I. (2007), 'Neuropsychological evidence for a strategic control of multiple routes in imitation'. *Brain*, 130, 4, pp. 1111–1126.

Tessitore, G., Sinigaglia, C., Prevete, R. (2013), 'Hierarchical and multiple hand action representation using temporal postural synergies'. *Experimental Brain Research*, 225, 1, pp. 11–36.

Tkach, D., Reimer, J., Hatsopoulos, N.G. (2007), 'Congruent activity during action and action observation in motor cortex'. *Journal of Neuroscience*, 27, 48, pp. 13241–13250.

Tomeo, E., Cesari, P., Aglioti, S.M., Urgesi, C. (2013), 'Fooling the kickers but not the goalkeepers: Behavioral and neurophysiological correlates of fake action detection in soccer'. *Cerebral Cortex*, 23, 11, pp. 2765–2778.

Tracey, I., Mantyh, P.W. (2007), 'The cerebral signature for pain perception and its modulation'. *Neuron*, 55, 3, pp. 377–391.

Tranel, D., Kemmerer, D., Adolphs, R., Damasio, H., Damasio, A.R. (2003), 'Neural correlates of conceptual knowledge for actions'. *Cognitive Neuropsychology*, 20, 3–6, pp. 409–432.

Tremblay, L., Worbe, Y., Thobois, S., Sgambato-Faure, V., Féger, J. (2015), 'Selective dysfunction of basal ganglia subterritories: From movement to behavioral disorders'. *Movement Disorders: Official Journal of the Movement Disorder Society*, 30, 9, pp. 1155–1170.

Trevarthen, C. (1998), 'The concept and foundations of infant intersubjectivity'. In *Intersubjective Communication and Emotion in Early Ontogeny*, Bråten, S. (editor), Cambridge University Press, Cambridge, UK, pp. 15–46.

Tucker, M., Ellis, R. (1998), 'On the relations between seen objects and components of potential actions'. *Journal of Experimental Psychology: Human Perception and Performance*, 24, 3, pp. 830–846.

Tucker, M., Ellis, R. (2001), 'The potentiation of grasp types during visual object categorization'. *Visual Cognition*, 8, 6, pp. 769–800.

Tucker, M., Ellis, R. (2004), 'Action priming by briefly presented objects'. *Acta Psychologica*, 116, 2, pp. 185–203.

Ulanovsky, N., Moss, C.F. (2007), 'Hippocampal cellular and network activity in freely moving echolocating bats'. *Nature Neuroscience*, 10, 2, pp. 224–233.

Umiltà, M.A., Kohler, E., Gallese, V., Fogassi, L., Fadiga, L., Keysers, C., Rizzolatti, G. (2001), 'I know what you are doing: A neurophysiological study'. *Neuron*, 32, pp. 91–101.

Umiltà, M.A., Escola, L., Intskirveli, I., Grammont, F., Rochat, M., Caruana, F., Jezzini, A., Gallese, V., Rizzolatti, G. (2008), 'When pliers become fingers in the monkey motor system'. *Proceedings of the National Academy of Sciences*, 105, 6, pp. 2209–2213.

Urgesi, C., Calvo-Merino, B., Haggard, P., Aglioti, S.M. (2007), 'Transcranial magnetic stimulation reveals two cortical pathways for visual body processing'. *Journal of Neuroscience*, 27, 30, pp. 8023–8030.

Urgesi, C., Candidi, M., Ionta, S., Aglioti, S.M. (2007), 'Representation of body identity and body actions in extrastriate body area and ventral premotor cortex'. *Nature Neuroscience*, 10, 1, pp. 30–31.

Urgesi, C., Savonitto, M.M., Fabbro, F., Aglioti, S.M. (2012), 'Long-and short-term plastic modeling of action prediction abilities in volleyball'. *Psychological Research*, 76, 4, pp. 542–560.

Vaca, G.F.B., Lüders, H.O., Basha, M.M., Miller, J.P. (2011), 'Mirth and laughter elicited during brain stimulation'. *Epileptic Disorders*, 13, 4, pp. 435–440.

Van Der Meer, A.L. (1997), 'Keeping the arm in the limelight: Advanced visual control of arm movements in neonates'. *European Journal of Paediatric Neurology*, 1, 4, pp. 103–108.

Van Der Meer, A.L., Van Der Weel, F., Lee, D. (1995), 'The functional significance of arm movements in neonates'. *Science*, 267, 5198, pp. 693–695.

Van Kemenade, B.M., Muggleton, N., Walsh, V., Pinar Saygin, A. (2012), 'Effects of TMS over premotor and superior temporal cortices on biological motion perception'. *Journal of Cognitive Neuroscience*, 24, 4, pp. 896–904.

Venkatraman, A., Edlow, B.L., Immordino-Yang, M.H. (2017), 'The brainstem in emotion: A review'. *Frontiers in Neuroanatomy*, 11, p. 15.

Viaro, R., Maggiolini, E., Farina, E., Canto, R., Iriki, A., D'Ausilio, A., Fadiga, L. (2021), 'Neurons of rat motor cortex become active during both grasping execution and grasping observation'. *Current Biology*, 31, 19, pp. 4405–4412.

Vigneswaran, G., Philipp, R., Lemon, R.N., Kraskov, A. (2013), 'M1 corticospinal mirror neurons and their role in movement suppression during action observation'. *Current Biology*, 23, 3, pp. 236–243.

Vignolo, L.A., Boccardi, E., Caverni, L. (1986), 'Unexpected CT-scan findings in global aphasia'. *Cortex*, 22, pp. 55–69.

Vogt, B.A. (2005), 'Pain and emotion interactions in subregions of the cingulate gyrus'. *Nature Reviews Neuroscience*, 6, 7, pp. 533–544.

Vogt, B.A., Berger, G.R., Derbyshire, S.W. (2003), 'Structural and functional dichotomy of human mincingulate cortex'. *European Journal of Neuroscience*, 18, 11, pp. 3134–3144.

Vogt, B.A., Sikes, R.W. (2009), 'Cingulate nociceptive circuitry and roles in pain processing: The cingulate premotor pain model'. In *Cingulate Neurobiology and Disease*, Vogt, B.A. (editor), Oxford University Press, New York, pp. 311–338.

Von Hofsten, C. (2004), 'An action perspective on motor development'. *Trends in Cognitive Science*, 8, 6, pp. 266–272.

Vrticka, P., Black, J.M., Reiss, A.L. (2013), 'The neural basis of humour processing'. *Nature Reviews Neuroscience*, 6, 7, pp. 533–544.

Wager, T.D., Atlas, L.Y., Lindquist, M.A., Roy, M., Woo, C.W, Kross, E. (2013), 'An fMRI-based neurologic signature of physical pain'. *New England Journal of Medicine*, 368, pp. 1388–1397.

Waxman, S.G. (1996), 'Clinical observations on the emotional motor system'. *Progress in Brain Research*, 107, pp. 595–604.

Webb, A., Knott, A., MacAskill, M.R. (2010), 'Eye movements during transitive action observation have sequential structure'. *Acta Psychologica*, 133, 1, pp. 51–56.

Weissensteiner, J., Abernethy, B., Farrow, D., Müller, S. (2008), 'The development of anticipation: A cross-sectional examination of the practice experiences contributing to skill in cricket batting'. *Journal of Sport and Exercise Psychology*, 30, 6, pp. 663–684.

Wicker, B., Keysers, C., Plailly, J., Royet, J.P., Gallese, V., Rizzolatti, G. (2003), 'Both of us disgusted in my insula: The common neural basis of seeing and feeling disgust'. *Neuron*, 40, pp. 655–664.

Witt, J.K., Proffitt, D.R., Epstein, W. (2005), 'Tool use affects perceived distance, but only when you intend to use it'. *Journal of Experimental Psychology: Human Perception and Performance*, 31, 5, pp. 880–888.

Witt, J.K., Proffitt, D.R. (2008), 'Action-specific influences on distance perception: A role for motor simulation'. *Journal of Experimental Psychology: Human Perception and Performance*, 34, 6, pp. 1479–1492.

Wohlschläger, A. (2000), 'Visual motion priming by invisible actions'. *Vision Research*, 40, 8, pp. 925–930.

Wohlschläger, A. (2001), 'Mental object rotation and the planning of hand movements'. *Perception and Psychophysics*, 63, 4, pp. 709–718.

Wood, A., Rychlowska, M., Korb, S., Niedenthal, P. (2016), 'Fashioning the face: Sensorimotor simulation contributes to facial expression recognition'. *Trends in Cognitive Sciences*, 20, 3, pp. 227–240.

Woodward, A.L. (1998), 'Infants selectively encode the goal object of an actor's reach'. *Cognition*, 69, 1, pp. 1–34.

Woodward, A.L. (1999), 'Infants' ability to distinguish between purposeful and non-purposeful behaviors'. *Infant Behavior and Development*, 22, 2, pp. 145–160.

Woodward, A.L., Gerson, S.A. (2014), 'Mirroring and the development of action understanding'. *Philosophical Transactions of the Royal Society B: Biological Sciences*, 369, 1644, 20130181.

Woolley, J.D., Strobl, E.V., Sturm, V.E., Shany-Ur, T., Poorzand, P., Grossman, S., Nguyen, L., Eckart, J.A., Levenson, R.W., Seeley, W.W., Miller, B.L., Rankin, K.P. (2015), 'Impaired recognition and regulation of disgust is associated with distinct but partially overlapping patterns of decreased gray matter volume in the ventroanterior insula'. *Biological Psychiatry*, 78, 7, pp. 505–514.

Wright, M.J., Bishop, D.T., Jackson, R.C., Abernethy, B. (2010), 'Functional MRI reveals expert-novice differences during sport-related anticipation'. *NeuroReport*, 21, 2, pp. 94–98.

Yamao, Y., Matsumoto, R., Kunieda, T., Shibata, S., Shimotake, A., Kikuchi, T., Satow, T., Mikuni, N., Fukuyama, H., Ikeda, A., Miyamoto, S. (2015), 'Neural correlates of mirth and laughter: A direct electrical cortical stimulation study'. *Cortex*, 66, pp. 134–140.

Yoshida, K., Saito, N., Iriki, A., Isoda, M. (2011), 'Representation of others' action by neurons in monkey medial frontal cortex'. *Current Biology*, 21, 3, pp. 249–253.

Young, A., Perrett, D., Calder, A., Sprengelmeyer, R., Ekman, P. (2002), *Facial Expressions of Emotion: Stimuli and Tests (FEEST)*. Thames Valley Test Company, Bury St. Edmunds.

ANALYTICAL INDEX

For the benefit of digital users, indexed terms that span two pages (e.g., 52–53) may, on occasion, appear on only one of those pages.

Figures are indicated by *f* following the page number